Stress and Pregnancy

Stress in Modern Society: No. 8

Other Titles in This Series:

No. 1. James H. Humphrey, ed. *Stress in Childhood,* 1984.

No. 2. James H. Humphrey. *Profiles in Stress,* 1986.

No. 3. Joy N. Humphrey and James H. Humphrey. *Coping with Stress in Teaching,* 1986.

No. 4. George S. Everly, Jr. and Stephen A. Sobelman. *Assessment of the Human Stress Response,* 1987.

No. 6. Jerrold S. Greenberg. *Stress and Sexuality.* 1987.

No. 12 Amarjit S. Sethi. *Meditation As an Intervention in Stress Reactivity.* 1989.

No. 13. Judity L. Hanna. *Dance and Stress: A Holistic Approach to Dealing with Stress.* 1988.

No. 16. M. Lawrence Furst and Donald R. Morse. *The Woman's World.* 198 .

No. 17. Donald R. Morse and Robert L. Pollack. *Nutrition, Stress, and Aging: An Holistic Approach.* 1988.

No. 18. James H. Humphrey. *Children and Stress: Theoretical Perspectives and Recent Research.* 1988.

No. 19. Donald R. Morse and Robert L. Pollack. *The Stress-Free, Anti-Aging Diet.* 1989.

STRESS IN MODERN SOCIETY
Number 8

Stress and Pregnancy

John Sullivan
and
Joyce Cameron Foster

AMS PRESS, INC.
New York

Library of Congress Cataloging in Publication Data

Sullivan, John J., 1919-
Stress and pregnancy.

(Stress in modern society; no. 8)
Includes index.
1. Stress (Psychology) 2. Pregnant women—Mental health.
3. Pregnant women—Psychological testing.
I. Foster, Joyce Cameron. II. Title. III. Series.
[DNLM: 1. Pregnancy—psychology. 2. Stress, Psychological. WQ 200 S949s]
RG580.S73S85 1989 618.3 86-82022
ISBN 0-404-63261-0

All AMS books are printed on acid-free paper that meets the guidelines for performance and durability of the Committee on Production Guidelines for Book Longevity of the Council on Library Resources.

AMS Press, Inc.
56 East 13th Street
New York, N.Y. 10003

MANUFACTURED IN THE UNITED STATES OF AMERICA

CONTENTS

— About the Authors:

John Sullivan, Ph.D. is currently a Research Associate in the Department of Surgery of the College of Medicine of the University of Utah. He was formerly a Research Professor at the College of Nursing at the University of Utah. Trained originally as an experimental psychologist (learning) his current interests are in the multivariate analysis of health and medical problems. He obtained a B.A. at the University of Minnesota, and a Ph.D. at the University of Iowa. He taught for many years in the Department of Educational Psychology at New York University.

Joyce Cameron Foster, Ph.D., RN, CNM is currently Associate Professor of Nursing and Director of the Graduate Nurse-Midwifery Program in the College of Nursing at the University of Utah. Her major research, teaching, and clinical focus is on development of high level wellness in childbearing women and their families through study of relevent variables, preparation of certified nurse-midwives qualified to foster high level wellness in their clients, and application of research in practice. She obtained her B.S. in Nursing at the University of California at Los Angeles, her Master of Science in Nursing and preparation in Nurse-Midwifery at Yale University, and her Ph.D. in Health Science at the University of Utah.

PREFACE

The work presented here is a result of the expert and dedicated effort of many individuals. We owe a not small debt to Phillip Merrifield, PhD of New York University whose experience in psychological measurement helped to set us on the course of action we took to develop the PIPAS (Pregnancy, Illness Proneness, and Stress) scales. His highly developed research problem solving skills were invaluable. Dr. Thomas H. Holmes, of the Department of Psychiatry and Behavioral Sciences of the School of Medicine of the University of Washington graciously gave us permission to use some items from the *Schedule of Experience (SRE)* in our stress scales. Without the groundbreaking work of Drs. Holmes and Rahe, we would not have developed our own research program.

We wish to acknowledge the contributions of Sally Yeomans, MSN, RN, CNM, and Margie Freston, PhD, RN, CNM for their clinical insights into the development of the pregnancy symptom scales and stress items. The support and effort of the nurses who administered the PIPAS scales to their childbirth classes during their development and refinement is much appreciated. We wish to thank Yvonne Caroles, RN, Esther Anderson, MS, RN, CNM, Donna Woolsey, RN, and Nancy Bolles, MS, RN, CNM, and Ann Marie Faxel, MS, RN, CNM for facilitating the use of childbirth classes at MacKay-Dee hospital, LDS Hospital, St. Marks Hospital, and the Phoenix Memorial Hospital respectively. A valuable contribution was made by Roselyn Darling, who served as a research assistant for data analyses during the initial development of the PIPAS scales. We appreciate the work of Carol Kirgis, PhD RN, who contributed to the research in the early phase of the project with her study predicting infant Apgar Scores.

A number of graduate students used the scales and/or the data in their master's theses at the University of Utah College of Nursing. Particular mention should be made of the excellent contribution of Sister Deborah Fuchs, who established the reliability and validity of the father data of the *Utah Test for the Childbearing Year*. Her thesis and those of the other graduate students are listed in Appendix F. The nurse-midwifery students at the College of Nursing who have taught the Childbearing Year Program as a part of their graduate work, through their use of the scales and feedback to us regarding the couples responses to both the assessment and teaching program, have contributed to our knowledge and understanding of stress in pregnancy. The contributions of two former students of psychology and measurement, Nancy Fagley and Paul Miller, are noted with appreciation.

This program of research has been supported by P.H.S. Grant MC-R490355, March of Dimes Grants CHE-34/11/32 and CHE-33/11-54, and Department of HEW Division of Nursing Grant NU 28028. Without the financial support and encouragement of these agencies we could not have conducted the research. Their assistance is appreciated.

Special thanks and appreciation are owed to Michelle Wright, who served as secretary during all of the grant periods, administered the many activities relative to the projects, and became a valued research assistant. She developed and carried out the procedures whereby the scales are packaged and given to the expectant parents, profiles are prepared, and data are recorded for use in the Childbearing Year program. Without her cheerful attention to numerous details, we could not have accomplished our work.

Finally, we wish to mention the gratification we have each received through our mutual association as colleagues over a number of years. The collaboration of our different professional interests and backgrounds, the respect we share for each other's ability to bring a unique focus to our research, and the shared pleasure in the outcome of each step have been valued experiences.

John Sullivan had the primary responsibility for drafting Chapters 1 and 2. Joyce Foster drafted Chapters 3 and 4. The authors jointly reviewed and edited all chapters as well as writing the Introduction and Summary.

INTRODUCTION

Human pregnancy presents a unique state in which the phenomenon of stress may be examined. Pregnancy is a time-limited experience in which there are enormous physical and physiological adjustments and changes (stresses). As the fetus grows and puts an increasing physiological load on the pregnant woman, the pregnancy process constitutes a "natural stress experiment." In addition, there is the experiential response of the woman and her partner. The amount of psychological stress during the pregnancy experience is a function of many factors: (a) personal, family, and cultural beliefs, perceptions, and expectations; (b) prior response patterns to stress and illness; (c) the extent of life stresses currently/recently experienced; (d) perceived and actual coping abilities; and (e) response to the physical/physiological changes of pregnancy. The vulnerability of the human organism to symptoms/illness during the pregnancy process is probably related to the total load of both physical and psychological stress. At the very least, the quality of the pregnancy experience is affected.

This monograph reports the development of a stress model and its use during pregnancy. Over a period of several years, we developed two batteries of scales, each with its relevant items reflecting the clinically appropriate psychological aspects of stress in pregnancy. One is the Pregnancy, Illness Proneness, and Stress (PIPAS) battery, and the other is the Utah Test for the Childbearing Year.

Stress, as we have defined it, is not limited to a single definition or conceptualization. Stress may be inferred in three ways: (a) by noting the conditions or situations the person is in, (b) by noting the individual's physiological condition and responses, and (c) by noting the individual's overt behavior. These three ways of viewing stress are referred to as $stress_1$, which is stimulus inferred; $stress_2$, which is physiologically inferred; and $stress_3$, which is response inferred by two process: (a) by reports of overt behavior, and (b) by interpreting the verbal (cognitive) self reports of an individual. The PIPAS scales are $stress_1$ measures; the Utah Test for the Childbearing Year, are $stress_3$ measures. An assay of the white blood count or catecholamine titre are examples of $stress_2$ measures.

The major battery of scales, PIPAS, is based on a central set of ideas on stress and illness proneness in general, applied to the course and outcomes of pregnancy. The basic hypothesis is that stress interacts with illness proneness with the result that stress activates illness prone tendencies. We conceptualize a continuum from extreme stress, which could be life threatening, to high-level wellness. Increased stress reduces wellness; high-level wellness reduces stress. In the case of the pregnant woman we expect that stress and illness-prone tendencies would be reflected in the number of symptoms the woman reported during pregnancy. We expect that the highly stressed and symptom-prone expectant mother would have a more difficult time and different outcomes than her lowly stressed and symptom-resistant counterpart.

Based originally on the work of Holmes and Rahe (1967) on adaptive strain, the PIPAS studies have evolved into a set of measures which assess: (a) symptom-proneness prior to pregnancy; (b) six scales for the measurement of stress in the areas of Family, Work, Social, Financial, Lifestyle, and Personal Habits Changes; and (c) six pregnancy symptoms scales for the measurement of Gastrointestinal, Reproductive, Neuromuscular, Skin, and Cardiovascular-Respiratory system symptoms, and General Adaptational Distress. In addition we have used the 20 psychiatric items of the Cornell Medical Index (Cornell Psychiatric Index or CPI).

The second battery of scales, The Utah Test for the Childbearing Year, was designed to measure cognitive beliefs and perceptions in five domains: (a) fear of the childbirth process, (b) childbirth health locus of control, (c) personal value about childbearing and childrearing, (d) passive compliance versus active participation in childbirth care decisions, and (e) the father's role and responsibility in childbearing. We hypothesize that beliefs and perceptions affect the woman's health in two ways: first, through her health behaviors, and, second, through physiologic manifestations or her fears and anxieties. Information from both of these batteries of scales may be readily assessed by using a paper and pencil questionnaire and correlated with other variables of interest.

The final step in our program of research has been to develop a system of clinical care that minimizes the stresses of pregnancy. We attempt to accomplish this through a comprehensive childbirth education program titled The Childbearing Year. The use of the scales in assessing the stress profile of the expectant couples and the elements of the program that relate to stress reduction and stress management during pregnancy are described. The stress reduction approach we are currently taking involves: (a) reducing physiologic stress through an individualized nutrition prescription, encouragement of a graded program of aerobic activity, use of effective body mechanics, muscle toning exercises, and specific techniques to reduce/control common physical discomforts and problems; (b) obtaining cognitive control over the events of pregnancy through specific information concerning the processes of pregnancy, birth and parenting; (c) understanding the stress phenomenon by providing feedback to each individual based on their own stress profile, followed by group discussion of specific information about stress and the value of stress reduction during pregnancy; and (d) reducing situational stresses and/or the intensity of response to unavoidable stresses, through application of a variety of specific strategies.

We believe that the concepts and scales presented in this monograph will be of interest and value not only to the researcher but to the clinician who is committed to the reduction of stress and the promotion of high-level wellness during childbearing and childrearing. We invite your use of these copyrighted scales either in research or practice.

References

Kirgis, C.A., Woolsey, D.B., & Sullivan, J.J. (1977). Predicting infant apgar scores. *Nursing Research, 26,* 6, 439-442.

Holmes, T.H. & Rahe, R.H. (1967). The social readjustment rating scale. *Journal of Psychosomatic Research, 11,* 213.

1

Stress And Pregnancy: Theory And Development Of The PIPAS Scales

Introduction

The PIPAS project is the name of a research program titled Ante-Peri- and Post-Natal Illness Proneness and Stress. The title is an acronym for Pregnancy, Illness Proneness, and Stress. Because the PIPAS project was fairly well funded, we were able to develop and to test by a series of studies a central set of ideas on stress and symptom proneness applied to the course and outcomes of pregnancy. In this chapter we describe both the conceptual orientation that gave the series of researches their coherence and the development of the various scales used in the PIPAS Project.

Our conceptual orientation, as the psychoanalysts would say, was overdetermined. That is, there were several strands of thought that led to the preliminary formulations, each of which could provide a sufficient rationale for the work. We mention briefly only two of these strands: (a) measurement of stress and the relations of these measures to illnesses as reported by T.H. Holmes (1967, 1970) and R.H. Rahe (1967-1972) and (b) studies on illness proneness.

Rahe (1972) summed up admirably the research on the *Schedule of Recent Experience* (SRE) in his review article in the *Annals of Clinical Research.* We include only the highlights of this review as it bore on the formulation of the rationale of the PIPAS project.

A number of investigators have compared the relationship of stress to illnesses. Others have studied the relation of events in the social lives of patients that were antecedent to illnesses. Holmes, Rahe (1967) and their collaborators have combined in one measure sets of critical social situations and an estimate of their stressful nature.

The basic strategy of their research has been (a) to identify a broad spectrum of significant life changes in individuals which preceded respiratory illnesses, (b) to scale these changes in terms of values of life change units and to call the resultant instrument the SRE, (c) to perform a series of similar scaling studies with different sub-groups in the United States and a few cross-cultural groups, (d) to conduct retrospective studies of life changes associated with illness, and finally (e) to make predictive studies of illnesses in which the predictor was the SRE scores. An outcome of these researches, Rahe reports, is that quantitative estimates can be given to the intensity of change inherent in life change events; and these Life Change Unit (LCU) experiences, when above 300 per year, have been shown to be clearly related to the probability of an individual becoming ill in the near future.

Development of PIPAS Theory

One of the starting points of our thinking on the problems of stress and illness was as follows: Let us assume that the SRE is a perfect measuring scale. It is a gratuitous assumption that the SRE is a perfect measuring scale because some of the failures to predict illnesses may well be due to the reliability level of the instrument. However, it was found that in one study 70% of those persons who had a yearly total of LCU over 300 would experience some illness in the near future. This finding is remarkable, but the 30% who were highly stressed yet did not report illnesses constitute a scientific anomaly. In addition, it seemed to us that some persons became ill who are not highly stressed. We thought that the stress/illness paradigm needed to be reformulated. These two conditions could be accounted for mathematically by the assumption of at least one other variable as a determinant of illnesses. We made this assumption and called the variable "illness proneness" (IP). If stress and illness-proneness were operating jointly, then we could expect a highly stressed individual who did not become ill to be illness-resistant, and a lowly stressed individual who did become ill to be illness-prone. Stress, however, would undoubtedly affect these resistant individuals, and they might become more neurotic, psychotic, or simply work harder compulsively. Similarly, we might expect some illness-prone persons to report many symptoms even though not very stressed.

Development of Stress Scales

To test our theoretical formulation, we decided to conduct a large-scale study on the relation of stress and illness proneness/illness resistance to the course and outcome of pregnancy. We first thought of using as a measure of stress the Life Change Units (LCU) scores as indexed by the Schedule of Recent Experience (SRE). Our admiration for the SRE, which we considered a genuine breakthrough in the measurement of stress, was great, but it was not unbounded. Although we were aware of some of its psychometric shortcomings, we used it as a means of entry into the problems of measurement of stress and pregnancy outcomes.

As soon as we were funded, we called in Phillip Merrifield of New York University as a consultant on our measurement problems. Dr. Merrifield is a specialist in psychological measurement, esteemed for his highly developed research problem-solving skills. We reviewed with him our general theory that stress activates illness-prone tendencies and that this process should be observable in the frequencies and intensities of normal and possibly high-risk symptoms during pregnancy, labor, and delivery. Because our behavioral science approach to the course of the pregnancy cycle was not characteristic of the usual research in this field, we anticipated the necessity of developing a system of measures for the processes we were studying. We discussed with Dr. Merrifield the procedural options open to us. Our problem was whether we should stick with undimensional measures, which we had used in pilot studies, or take a factor analytic approach to the measurement of stress and symptoms, and develop multiple measures of these concepts. Because he recommended a factor analytic approach, we decided to factor analyze the SRE.

The SRE is a 42-item scale in which each item has been given a weight in terms of its average LCU score, as assessed by the norm population of the test. There are two standard measurement criteria which we applied to the SRE: (a) Is the test unidimensional, and (b) how adequate are the weights applied to each of the items?

The unidimensionality criterion raises the question of the legitimacy and meaningfulness of summing up the item weights to a single general index. That is, does it make sense to sum up into one index the items from such diverse situations as family, work, society at large, and personal habits? Is the procedure one in which the units added are comparable despite the apparent diversity of the situations in which they occur? On the face of it, it seems that the common denominator of interest is the LCU aspect of the different situations, so that what is really added is life change units and not stress situations.

The second and related question of the appropriateness of the weights of the particular items for different populations could be answered easily. The weights were derived from a sample of 400 Seattle residents who were a fairly good general population match. The weights seemed to be remarkably stable when cross-cultural populations of a similar socio-economic level to the norm group were surveyed. But the question is of the efficacy of the weights for items in a scale for subgroups that depart substantially from the norm group. It is known (Rahe, 1972) that the significance of some of the events for some subgroups, inner-city Los Angeles Chicanos, for example, varied considerably from the norm group weights. We believed that the Holmes and Rahe weights applied to intermountain pregnant women attending prenatal classes were inappropriate. In terms of life change units, most of them should have been seriously ill. At that period of life they customarily had been recently married, left school, started or stopped work, left their families to start new families, frequently borrowed money for a house or car, etc. In addition to all of these life changes, a profoundly significant one for a woman was being pregnant. Table 1 gives the life change units (LCU scores) for 116 pregnant women in a prenatal class at MacKay-Dee Hospital. The average LCU score was 410.922 with a standard deviation of 180.492. We suspected that the weights would have to be readjusted for our population of women. To rescale the weights of the test items for each population of interest is clearly a horrendous task that requires the original research to be done over again for each group studied.

Fortunately, there are good arguments and data, some of which we shall illustrate from our own research, indicating that a more flexible procedure than weighting items would be to develop subtests, and then by the use of regression equations to weight the subtests for each population and each particular dependent variable of interest.

TABLE 1

Schedule of Recent Experience Life Change Unit Scores Total for Year
N = 116
Women in prenatal class, McKay-Dee Hospital, Ogden, Utah (1974)

SRE Score	Frequency
0-100	4
101-200	15
201-300	22
301-400	26
401-500	27
501-600	11
601-700	4
701-800	4
801-900	1
901-1000	2
Total	116

Median	393.500
Mean	410.922
Standard Deviation	180.442
Kurtosis	.181
Skewness	.509

TABLE 2

Items By Factors When Loading is Greater Than .35
N = 116

Factor 1	Loading
Has there been a change in your financial state?	-.84
Have you changed your usual church activities?	-.81
Have you made any particular changes in your personal habits?	-.76
Have you been having either more or fewer arguments with your spouse?	-.68
Has there been a change in the number of your family get-togethers?	-.67
Have you had trouble wwith your in-laws?	-.67
Factor 2	
Have you had an increase in the number of people in your family?	-.90
Have you had a retirement from work?	-.88
Have you had trouble with your in-laws?	-.56
Have you been having either more or fewer arguments with your spouse?	-.54
Factor 3	
Have you had a change in the health of a family member?	-.94
Have you had any changes in your sleeping habits?	-.81
Have you experienced the death of a close friend?	-.81
Have you experienced the death of your spouse?	-.79
Have you been having sexual difficulties?	-.63
Factor 4	
Have you experienced a change in your responsibilities at work?	.60
Have you been on vacation?	.49
Have you been having sexual difficulties?	.45
Have you experienced a marital reconciliation?	.43
Have you gotten married?	.41
Have you had a business readjustment?	.36

Factor 5	Loading
Have you served a jail term?	.89
Have you gotten divorced?	.71
Have you changed the kind of recreation in which you usually engage?	.63
Have you changed to a difference line of work?	.51
Has your husband (or wife) begun or stopped working?	.42
Have you had a mortgage over $10,000?	.37

Factor 6	
Have you been fired at work?	-.71
Have you had any changes in your sleeping habits?	-.58
Have you experienced a change in living conditions?	-.53

Factor 7	
Have you been having sexual difficulties?	-.48
Have you had a mortgage for less than $10,000?	-.46
Have you experienced a foreclosure of a mortgage of loan?	-.46

Factor 8	
Have you changed your work hours or work conditions?	.52

Appears on No Factor

Do you have trouble with your boss?
Have you had any changes in your eating habits for better or worse?
Have you changed your usual social activities?
Have you had any personal injury or illness?
Have you had a change in residence?
Have you experienced the death of a close family member?
Have you been arrested for a minor violation of the law?
Have you experienced a marital separation for any reason?
Have you had some outstanding personal achievement?
Has your son or daughter left home?
Have you changed the school you attend?
Have you changed to a different line of work?
Have you had a pregnancy?

The present array of factor analytic options easily available in sets of programs is formidable. We decided to use the Biomedical Department (of UCLA) statistical package with the following parameters: (a) because the constraints on our test construction plans were that we could not have more than 5-7 scales of 20 items each, we programmed the computer to extract as many factors as possible, but to rotate only the first eight; (b) the communalities in the initial correlation matrix were to be filled by an iteration procedure; (c) the rotation of factors was to oblique axes by the Oblim method with a Gamma+ .5000. We had SRE scores on 103 subjects who were attending a prenatal class at MacKay-Dee Hospital for the factor analysis.

There were nine eigenvalues greater than 1.0, and the set of these factors accounted for 49% of the variance of the test. The factor loadings of the items on each of the factors is to be found in Table 2. With some misgivings we named the factors as follows:

Factor 1 — Living Style Stress (Stystr)
Factor 2 — Family Stress (Famstr)
Factor 3 — Personal Habits Stress (Perstr)
Factor 4 — Work Stress (Wkrstr)
Factor 5 — Social Norm Stress (Socstr)
Factor 6 — Not used
Factor 7 — Financial Stress (Finstr)
Factor 8 — Not used

We discovered that 13 items did not appear on any of the first eight factors. This means, in effect, that these items were contributing to random variance of the group that we were studying. These 13 items, although not in any scale, are important clinically. This is a good example of how a clinician must, in the assessment of any particular patient, supplement the use of standard scales by including items which are relevent but not in the scales. The factor analysis shows that many of the stress situations tend to covary in groups as indicated by the factors, but some situations that contribute to the total life change stresses are not associated with any of the major subgroups of items.

Using the names of the factors and the particular items found in the factor clusters we then constructed six scales of 28 items each. These 28 items were then reduced to 16 by looking at item means and standard deviations. We gave these scales to 202 women and item-analyzed each scale by means of the University of Wisconsin FORTAP program. This program gives α coefficient reliabilities and the point biserial correlation of each item with the total of the scale score. We selected the items having the highest correlation with the total scale scores. Table 3 gives the reliabilities of the scales and item-total correlations for a sample of 234 subjects.

As is well known, the reliabilities of scales vary with the number of items in the scale and the quality of the items. The reliabilities of these scales are good enough for research purposes and could be increased if we were to increase the number of items in each scale. However, we were under the constraint to limit the size of our scales to about 14-18 items per scale so that we could put other scales in our test battery. It is clear that the weakest scale is the Social Stress scale. As can be seen from Table 3, this scale has items which indicate some social disorganization, impulsivity, and social transgressions. For this particular group of persons, these items are not frequent, but when they do occur they must have some serious stress consequences. We are measuring Work Stress, Living Style Stress, and Personal Habits Changes Stress well so that we expect in future that these measures will be given appreciable weights in our regression equations.

The logic of our procedure rests on the assumption that the reliability of individual items is much less than the reliability of individual scales. How this works can be seen from an inspection of Table 3. Some items have a high item-total correlation within one time period and not in another. For instance, for this group of subjects for the 0-6 months ago interval of the item "Have you had a close friend who has been arrested or jailed?" in the Social Stress scale, the item-total is .800; but for the 6-12 months ago interval the item total correlation is .3689. Thus, this is a good Social Stress score item for this group during the 6-12 months period but not for the 0-6 months period. Even more indicative of how items change is the response to the item of the Personal Habits Changes Stress scale "Have you been a vegetarian?" Apparently, in the group upon which the items were selected the women with a history of vegetarianism were highly stressed. In this group either there were no vegetarians or some very tranquil vegetarians. For this group the item does not function at all.

TABLE 3

UTAH Stress Scales: Item Total Correlations and Scale Reliabilities

Scales	234 Subjects October 1975 0-6 Months Ago	234 Subjects October 1975 0-12 Months Ago
SOCSTR		
Total Scale Reliability	.4472	.4550
Have you been arrested for a minor violation?	.0813	.1093
Have you had a fight with a close friend?	.3955	.4987
Have you been either drunk or disorderly?	.3910	.4472
Have you left home for a period of hours or longer because of a dispute?	.4549	.3932
Have you changed marital partners?	.1299	.2760
Have you been abandoned by your family?	.1134	.0842
Have you run away from home?	.1681	.2099
Have you had a close friend who has been arrested or jailed?	.0800	.3689
Have you been planning any legal action against someone?	.4043	.2084
Have you occasionally used social drugs (marijuana, alcohol)?	.3329	.6139
Have you thought of suicide?	.2195	.2990
Have you been a victim of a swindle or fraud?	.2480	.2552
Have you been a victim of a serious crime?	.1299	.0000
Have you become fearful of being alone	.5276	.5031
while at home?		.0842
Have you gotten divorced?	.2706	
Have you exceeded the speed limit by more than 10 miles per hour?	.5128	.4759
WRKSTR		
Total Scale Reliability	.8014	.7288
Have you changed to a different line of work?	.4480	.4287
Have you had a change in responsibilities at work?	.6495	.3256
Have you had trouble with your boss?	.3502	.2401
Have you had a change in attitude towards your job?	.6696	.6164

Scales	234 Subjects October 1975 0-6 Months Ago	234 Subjects October 1975 0-12 Months Ago
WRKSTR *(continued)*		
Have you had a change in your boss?	.4928	.4540
Have you had a change in your co-workers?	.5530	.5009
Have you had a change in your physical conditions at work?	.4242	.3443
Have you had a change in your work due to seasonal changes?	.2468	.2780
Have you had a temporary change in the kind of work you do?	.4456	.4473
Have you had a change in work which strains your competencies	.4653	.1737
Have you had a change in work which now does does not make good use of your capacities?	.3463	.3817
Have you changed the location of your work?	.4760	.5586
Have you felt that your work has become more of a strain for you because of your pregnancy?	.4336	.4315
Have you changed your work hours or work conditions?	.5748	.5586
Have you strongly disliked your work?	.5097	.4565
Have your co-workers generally been satisfied with their work?	.4811	.5195
Have you wanted to quit your present job (if you could afford not to work)?	.6478	.4504
Do you tend to feel physically and emotionally	.5207	.5032
FAMSTR		
Total Scale Reliability	.6138	.6448
Have you had a change in your role as wife or mother?	.4171	.4267
Have you experienced a marital reconciliation?	.2794	.0964
Have you had a change in the number of family get-togethers?	.3191	.3840
Have you gotten married?	.4229	.3124
Have you had trouble with your in-laws?	.3006	.3152
Have you had more or fewer arguments with your spouse?	.5065	.3872

Scales	234 Subjects October 1975 0-6 Months Ago	234 Subjects October 1975 0-12 Months Ago
FAMSTR *(continued)*		
Have you had difficulties in your sexual relationship?	.4487	.5026
Have you discussed a possible separation from your spouse?	.4176	.3206
Have you had an increase or decrease in the number of people in your household?	.3850	.5789
Have you had religious conflicts within your household?	.4196	.4942
Have you had political or religious conflicts in your family?	.4353	.4057
Have you experienced the death of a close family member?	.1777	.2361
Have you experienced a change of attitude toward your family?	.5301	.4537
Have you had conflicts over who performs various tasks in your household?	.3711	.4174
Have you had arguments about family finances?	.3703	.4341
Have you had some outstanding personal achievement?	.3352	.2528
Have you had a pregnancy?	.2789	.4237
Has your family changed in any important way?	Missing	.3465
FINSTR		
Total Scale Reliability	.5217	.6292
Do you have a mortgage over $10,000?	.2591	.3815
Do you have a mortgage under $10,000?	.1570	.2273
Do you have monthly car payments?	.4278	.3879
Do you have a bank loan (other than education, house, or car loan)?	.2882	.3847
Do you have any outstanding medical bills?	.1604	.2428
Have you had a reduction in family income?	.3284	.2376
Have you had an increase in family income?	.1965	.5014
Have you had a change in your financial state?	.5141	.5091
Has recent inflation forced you to shop more carefully?	.5206	.5430

Scales	234 Subjects October 1975 0-6 Months Ago	234 Subjects October 1975 0-12 Months Ago
FINSTR *(continued)*		
Have you recently made a major purchase (house, furniture, car, etc.)?	.3476	.4360
Have you changed your food habits because of inflation?	.3694	.3431
If you have a checking account, have you overdrawn it?	.2806	.3314
Have you had to borrow money from your family or friends?	.3020	.4237
Have you put money away each month in a savings account?	.3279	.3116
Have you bought major purchases on credit?	.3061	.4270
Has there been a change in your financial state?	.4986	.4929
Have you had to change your vacation plans because of financial reasons?	.3307	.3389
LIVSTR		
Total Scale Reliability	.7657	.7809
Have you had a change in living conditions?	.5371	.6271
Have you had a change in residence?	.5058	.4821
Have you begun or finished school?	.3805	.4845
Have you had a change in your usual social activities?	.6171	.5385
Have you had a change in your usual church activities?	.4340	.3312
Have you started or stopped any social activities?	.5800	.6022
Have you had a difficult time budgeting for household expenses?	.3073	.4189
Have you had a change in your hobby?	.4074	.3643
Have you had a change in your mode of transportation?	.3369	.2518
Have you had a change more or less in the time you spend by yourself?	.6020	.5124
Have you felt that you never have enough time for yourself?	.3752	.3609
Have you been spending less time in outdoor activities?	.5146	.6457

Scales	234 Subjects October 1975 0-6 Months Ago	234 Subjects October 1975 0-12 Months Ago
LIVSTR *(continued)*		
Have you watched television or read more than before your pregnancy?	.4330	.4679
Have you changed from thinking of yourself as a pregnant woman to being the mother of an unborn baby?	.3019	.5303
Have you become close to or lost some friends?	.5392	.4149
Have you changed your style of dressing?	.4543	.5896
Have you changed your shopping habits?	.4648	.4645
Have you changed your hair style or cosmetic make-up?	Missing	.3143
PERSTR		
Total Scale Reliability	.7692	.7850
Have you changed some of your personal habits?	.4801	.5945
Have you changed some of your eating habits?	.4970	.5827
Have you changed some of your sleeping habits?	.5833	.5570
Have you changed some of your exercising habits?	.4822	.5644
Have you changed your recreational habits?	.5466	.5493
Have you been a vegetarian?	.0025	.0790
Have you gone on or off a reducing diet?	.1743	.3301
Have you changed the time you wake up or go to bed?	.6010	.4962
Have you had a change in the quality of your dreams?	.4620	.5115
Have you changed the amount of time you spend doing housework?	.4579	.5430
Have you increased or decreased activities in church?	.5102	.4557
Have you increased or decreased social contacts?	.5144	.5440
Have you seemed to feel more optimistic	.3489	.3130
Have you experienced considerable mood changes?	.5498	.5694
Have you had any personal injury or illness?	.2079	.1197
Have you had a change in your sex life?	.4922	.4358
Have you had a change in your daily activities?	.5395	.5415

Such are the vicissitudes of item reliabilities: why scales composed of many items tend to be more reliable than those composed of only a few items.

Frequencies and Intercorrelations of Stress Scales

Table 4 gives the means and standard deviations of each of the stress scales for 342 subjects who took the test in the late summer and early fall of 1975. It can be seen that the Social Stress scale which has the lowest reliability (Table 3) also has the fewest number of average responses, and the standard deviation of the distribution of scores almost equals the mean of the distribution. This indicates that the distribution is positively skewed. In general, as the reliability of the scales goes up, the average number of responses goes up, and the distribution of scores more nearly approaches normal. Note that, except for Work Stress, the number of positive responses to the stress reports for the 0-6 months ago interval is higher than the stress reports for the period from 6-12 months ago. We believe that this is partly a memory factor in that there is a decrement in

TABLE 4

Means and Standard Deviations of 342 Subjects

	0-6 Months Ago		6-12 Months Ago	
	Mean	Std. Dev.	Mean	Std. Dev.
1. SOCSTR	1.663	1.443	1.211	1.8655
2. WRKSTR	2.530	2.674	1.192	1.5805
3. FAMSTR	3.198	2.144	1.836	1.8815
4. FINSTR	4.280	2.688	2.788	2.193
5. STYSTR	4.657	2.995	2.181	2.3195
6. PERSTR	5,452	3.5775	1.859	2.3515
TOTAL	21.780		18.729	

the number of stresses when they are reported by a recall process. We find memory decrement also when we ask women who are in their second trimester to recall their symptoms during the first trimester. They seem to be able to recall the symptoms and stresses that they are actually feeling in greater number than those that they might have had some time ago. We shall report further studies on this tendency.

Table 5 gives the intercorrelations of the UTAH stress scales in two groups of subjects. As can be seen, the intercorrelation in each sample is approximately the same. Social Stress and Work Stress do not correlate highly with the other scales. Family Stress in one sample correlated moderately with Social Stress and with Personal Habits Changes Stress. Living Style Stress correlates with Family Stress, Financial Stress, and Personal Habits Changes Stress. It seems to us to be a general stress measure to which all of the other family, financial and personal stresses contribute. In regresion equations in which Family Stress, Financial Stress and Personal Habits Changes Stress have been entered, the Living Style Stress adds nothing to the prediction equation. We have a similar

TABLE 5

Utah Stress Scales Correlation Matrix 0-6 Months Ago

	1	2	3	4	5	6
1	—	.3913	.5109	.3992	.4522	.4621
2	.0373	—	.2949	.3032	.3709	.3547
3	.2983	.2483	—	.4650	.6340	.6118
4	.1910	.1159	.4300	—	.5064	.4875
5	.2182	.1576	.5419	.4626	—	.7438
6	.2644	.2026	.6308	.4026	.6919	—

Lower Triangle N = 140
Upper Triangle N = 202

phenomenon with our sets of symptoms scales, which we will only mention now but will discuss in more detail later. Among our six symptom scales, we have a set of symptoms that we call General Adaptational Distress. These symptoms have the highest correlation with all the other symptom groups, and it seems to us that the other symptoms contribute to this General Adaptational Distress in somewhat the same way that Family, Financial, and Personal Habits Changes Stress contribute to Living Style stress. We are not particularly happy with the fact that these two scales, General Adaptational Distress and Living Style Stress, correlate with the other scales, but it makes sense to us conceptually, even if these scales do not add much independent variance to our regression equations.

Comparison of Stress Scales with SRE

Having developed six scales with the properties given above, we raised the question as to how well these particular scales did in comparison with the SRE in predicting reports of symptoms during each of the trimesters. The results are in Table 6. The differences between the correlations is striking and is due to two factors that need some explanation.

As far as the SRE correlations are concerned there is no particular methodological difficulty. The person's SRE scores were simply correlated with the total number of symptoms reported during the particular trimester. But for the UTAH Stress scales the correlations were obtained in the following way: The scales were developed on the 202 cases by means of the item analysis discussed earlier. Then a separate regression equation was constructed for the total symptoms for each stress interval period — that is, the second trimester symptoms were the dependent variables for the total of the six stress scales during the 6-12 months period before taking the test and the multiple correlation was .44. Then the second trimester symptoms were the dependent variables in a regression equation in which the independent variables were the stress scores for the 0-6 months ago interval, and the multiple correlation was .50. Finally, the second trimester symptoms were the dependent variable and the independent variables were the 12 scores on the stress scales, 6 for the 6-12 months ago period and 6 for the 0-6 months ago period, and the multiple correlation was .58.

The undoubted superiority of the UTAH Stress Scales is due to two factors, one good and one not so good. The first factor is that our system is sensitive to the fact that each of the trimesters is almost a qualitatively

TABLE 6

Comparison of Correlations of Schedule of Recent Experience (SRE) Scores and PIPAS Stress Scores with Number of Symptoms Reported Each Trimester

	SRE (N-249)			Utah Stress Scales (N=202)		
Trimester	Months 12-6	Months 0-6	Months 0-12	Months 12-6	Months 0-6	Months 0-12
1	.15	.23	.27	.44	.50	.58
II	.25	.34	.37	.33	.41	.48
III	.32	.21	.34	.47	.44	.51

different physiological problem for the pregnant woman (data will be presented later). Thus the symptoms change, and their relations to predictors change. These changes can be accommodated by the procedure of constructing new regression equations for each trimester, and having the stress scales optimally weighted for each different physiological condition. The basic superiority of our measurement procedure is assigning weights to scales rather than to items. The not so good aspect of these correlation coefficients is that they are slightly inflated due to the fact that the scales were derived from subjects that we later used for the correlations and regression equations. However, when the sample sizes are over 200, the statistical errors of the correlation coefficients are of such a small order that the inflation of the regression equations is quite small. Our estimate from other work is that the equations would drop about .1. We have found that the reliabilities of the scales across samples is fairly steady.

We thus conclude that our scales have predictive properties generally on the order of the SRE or slightly better, that we can easily reweight the scales to fit different populations and different dependent variables, and that we finally have some indication of the particular pattern of stresses for any given pregnant woman.

Development of Index of Symptom Proneness:

Medical research on illness proneness has been summarized admirably by Thurlow (1967). An extract of Hinkle's work (1959) follows:

1) There is a positive relation between the:
   number of illness episodes and the variety of illnesses
   number of illness episodes and illness involving many symptoms
   number of illness episodes and greatest number of causes reported
   number of minor illnesses and the number of major illnesses
2) The illnesses of an individual cluster about a mean, but fluctuate with life situations.
   According to Engel and Schmale (1965):
3) Illness occurs not at times of great physical or environmental

stress, but when the individual feels he is not able to cope with his environment.

There is an obvious analogy between the concept of symptom proneness and the concept of accident proneness. The distribution of symptoms, illnesses, and accidents tend to be similar, and each reflects events distributed in a positively skewed distribution. Of great interest in this research are the marked differences between the illness-resistant person compared to the illness-prone individual. Hinkle (1959) reports that in practically every group studied, 25% of the people have half, or little more than half, of all illness episodes over the prime of life; another 25% have fewer than 10% of the episodes (p. 22).

Encouraged by the reports in the scientific literature, our first problem was to see whether such a Stress IR-IP model would fit the course and outcomes of pregnancy by attempting to develop a good measure of illness proneness/illness resistance. For some people theoretical formulations of a loose type come easily, but the worth of the formulations depends upon whether (a) there are practical coordinating definitions between the theoretical constructions and measuring operations of empirical concepts; (b) there are measures available, or that could be developed, for the empirical concepts; and (c) finally that reality and its processes somehow have a similar structure and process to that assumed in the model.

Our operational definition of illness-proneness and illness-resistance was simply a frequency count of the number of symptoms and illnesses a person reported from a list presented as having occurred over the last 10 years of their adult life. In the early, naive stage of our work we simply adopted the idea of illness proneness and constructed a 40-item scale slightly modified from a type used as a quick preliminary screening device by internal medicine physicians. Table 7 gives the results of the first use of this scale.

We quickly arrived at the position that the illness items were inappropriate for the course of pregnancy because we were primarily interested in minor pregnancy symptoms. We then eliminated eight illness items from the original scale and renamed the scale "Symptom Proneness" (SP). Since all of our major work was done with the SP scale, this scale is presented in Table 8.

Reports of Symptoms

The Symptom Checklist had an α coefficient reliability of .80 based upon 1315 PIPAS subjects. Table 7 gives the distribution of the reports of symptoms and the basic descriptive statistics as provided by the Statistical Package for the Social Sciences (SPSS) program FREQUENCIES. As can be seen, the average number of symptoms reported from this list was 12.828 with a standard deviation of 8.318. When the standard deviation so closely approaches the mean, the distribution is not normal but is positively skewed. The amount of skewness is indicated by the skewness index of .538, zero being a symmetrical distribution. The distribution was also slightly platykurtic with a kurtosis index less than zero (normal) with a value of -.457.

To get a rough idea of the utility of the distribution, we thought of splitting the distribution in terms of the upper 20% and lower 20% of women reporting symptoms. This figure was arrived at by the consideration that roughly 80% of babies are born without much difficulty. About 20% have some minor symptoms, and of these 10% have symptoms which require care. Of these, about 1-3% require intensive care. The women in the lower 20% of the distribution had over the last ten years an average of 2.5 symptoms on the checklist. Those in the upper 20% reported an average of 24.6 symptoms. If the first group is operationally defined as Symptom-Resistant and the second operationally defined as Symptom-Prone, then the Symptom-Prone reported 9.8 times as many symptoms as the Symptom-Resistant. The Symptom Proneness items are listed in Table 8.

Cornell Psychiatric Items (CPI)

Our first-stage theory was that stress and symptom proneness interacted with and affected the minor symptoms of pregnancy. The next stage conceptualization quickly occurred. It was that the effects of stress and symptom proneness on the course of pregnancy were not only direct but also indirect through psychological upset. There are many indices of psychological disturbances such as the Minnesota Multiphasic Personality

TABLE 7

Reports of Symptoms
N = 116
Women in prenatal class, McKay Dee Hospital, Ogden, Otah (1974)

Number of Symptoms	Frequency
0 - 5	24
6 - 10	29
11 - 15	24
16 - 20	14
21 - 25	15
26 - 30	7
31 - 35	2
36 - 40	1
Total	116
Median	11.833
Mean	12.828
Standard Deviation	8.318
Kurtosis	-.457
Skewness	.538

TABLE 8

PIPAS Symptom Proneness Items

INSTRUCTIONS: Please circle the illnesses or symptoms you have had within the past ten years.

Example:

1. Gas
2. Stomach cramps
3. Gallbladder trouble
4. Hemorrhoids (piles)
5. Crampy pain in abdomen
6. Trouble with teeth/gums

TABLE 8 *(continued)*

This means you have had stomach cramps, hemorrhoids (piles), and a crampy pain in your abdomen within the past ten years, but have not had gas, gallbladder trouble or trouble with teeth/gums.

Remember: If the item is not applicable, you make no mark on the sheet. Please circle the illnesses or symptoms you have had within the past ten years.

1. Gas
2. Stomach cramps
3. Gallbladder trouble
4. Hemorrhoids (piles)
5. Crampy pain in abdomen
6. Trouble with teeth/gums
7. Loss of appetite for more than a day
8. Burning sensation in stomach
9. Sensitive to particular food
10. Earaches
11. Trouble with eyes
12. Prolonged stuffy nose
13. Severe headaches
14. Hay fever
15. Tonsillitis
16. Persistent cold in chest
17. Urinary tract infections
18. Bladder infections
19. Blood in urine
20. High or low blood pressure
21. Anemia
22. Bleeding tendency
23. Allergies
24. Chest pains
25. Persistent cough
26. Feeling of general weakness
27. Gain or loss of weight (more than 10%)
28. Severe menstrual cramps
29. Stiff or sore joints
30. Specific muscle weakness
31. Cuts or wounds which healed slowly
32. Bruise easily

α coefficient based upon 1315 pregnant women is: $\alpha = .80$

Inventory) and the CPI (California Personality Inventory), but we wanted a short scale designed to indicate rather severe psychological disorder. Whereas our battery of tests already included stress measures and a symptom proneness measure, and we were also going to develop minor pregnancy symptom scales, the psychological upset index had to be short. We selected the 20 psychiatric items of the Cornell Medical Index (1949). These items are given in Table 9.

Minor Pregnancy Symptom Scales

These scales were constructed in our usual fashion. We anticipated the development of five or six scales of approximately 12-15 items. To achieve this we developed six scales of about 25 items each, based upon the areas of inquiry used by nurse-midwives in their prenatal care of pregnant women. These scales were then given to pregnant women, and the final set of items were chosen on the basis of (a) high-point biserial correlation of an item with the total score of the test, and (b) response to the item by at least 10% of the women, and (c) moderate to large standard deviation of scales when ranked by standard deviations. The scales, with their reliabilities for each trimester, are given in Table 10. The intercorrelations are given in Table 11, and the correlations of the items with Symptom Proneness are given in Table 12.

The PIPAS battery of tests went through four versions in its development, and a final version which consisted of shortening the symptom and stress scale for the best nine items in each scale. We were lucky to be both well-funded and to have access to Utah's outstanding population sub-group, pregnant women. We were under constant pressure from clinicians to reduce the size of our battery to the sub-set of best items. Eventually, this is what we did. The final short form of the scales is in Appendix A.

In the next chapter we report on two of our many major studies. In these studies the short form of the scales was used, and we did not discriminate between types of stress or types of pregnancy symptoms.

TABLE 9

Psychiatric Items of the Cornell Medical Index Used in the PIPAS UTAH-IVS Format

Please circle the period(s) during THIS pregnancy in which you OFTEN had or are having any of the following symptoms.

		WHEN 1-3 MONTHS PREGNANT	WHEN 4-6 MONTHS PREGNANT	WHEN 7-9 MONTHS PREGNANT
1.	Did/do you get nervous and shaky when approached by someone you consider to be important?	Y	Y	Y
2.	Did/do you usually feel unhappy and depressed?	Y	Y	Y
3.	Did/does life look entirely hopeless?	Y	Y	Y
4.	Did/do you suffer from severe nervous exhaustion?	Y	Y	Y
5.	Did/does every little thing get on your nerves lately and wear you out?	Y	Y	Y
6.	Did/do you often become suddenly scared for no good reason?	Y	Y	Y
7.	Did/do you often wish you were dead and away from it all?	Y	Y	Y
8.	Did/does your thinking get completely mixed up when you have to do things quickly?	Y	Y	Y
9.	Were/are you constantly keyed up and jittery?	Y	Y	Y

TABLE 9

Psychiatric Items of the Cornell Medical Index Used in the PIPAS UTAH-IVS Format

		WHEN 1-3 MONTHS PREGNANT	WHEN 4-6 MONTHS PREGNANT	WHEN 7-9 MONTHS PREGNANT
10.	Did/do frightening thoughts keep coming back in your mind?	Y	Y	Y
11.	Did/do you often get spells of complete exhaustion or fatigue?	Y	Y	Y
12.	Were/are you often bothered by thumping of the heart?	Y	Y	Y
13.	Did/do you wear yourself out worrying about your health?	Y	Y	Y
14.	Did/does your heart often race like mad?	Y	Y	Y
15.	Did/does pressure or pain in the head often make life miserable for you?	Y	Y	Y

TABLE 9

Psychiatric Items of the Cornell Medical Index Used in the PIPAS UTAH-IVS Format

		WHEN 1-3 MONTHS PREGNANT	WHEN 4-6 MONTHS PREGNANT	WHEN 7-9 MONTHS PREGNANT
16.	Did/do you wish you always had someone at your side to advise you?	Y	Y	Y
17.	Did/do you go to pieces if you don't constantly control yourself?	Y	Y	Y
18.	Did/do you often shake or tremble?	Y	Y	Y
19.	Did/does worrying continually get you down?	Y	Y	Y
20.	Were/are you considered to be a nervous person?	Y	Y	Y

Number of cases = 1330
Alpha for first trimester = .787
Number of cases = 1354
Alpha for second trimester = .837
Number of cases = 703
Alpha for third trimester = .877

TABLE 10

Reliabilities of the Symptoms Scales

	# Items	Alpha Coefficient by Trimester		
		I	II	III
1. GI Gastro-Intestinal Symptoms	12	.66	.67	.80
2. GAD Symptoms of General Adaptational Distress	12	.70	.76	.87
3. REPR Reproductive System Symptoms	14	.53	.76	.53
4. NM Neuro-Muscular Symptoms	10	.51	.57	.81
5. SKIN Skin Symptoms	9	.39	.50	.70
6. CVR Cardio-Vascular-Respiratory Symptoms	13	.58	.69	.78
Total Symptoms	89	.88	.93	.97
Number of Cases		436	.407	152

TABLE 11

Utah Stress Scales
Correlation Matrix
12-6 Months Ago

	1	2	3	4	5	6
1.	—	.2877	.4349	.0478	.3196	.2929
2.	.0354	—	.3723	.2255	.4324	.4299
3.	.2248	.3616	—	.4308	.5634	.4941
4.	.1629	.2264	.4096	—	.4810	.4330
5.	.1177	.3629	.5938	.5437	—	.7484
6.	.1602	.3942	.6724	.4807	.7654	—

Lower Triangle N = 140
Upper Triangle N = 202

TABLE 12

Product-Moment Correlation of Illness Proneness/Resistance Index with Pregnancy Symptom Indices

	First Trimester (1) N = 436		Second Trimester N = 407		Third Trimester N = 152	
	IP with Symptoms		IP with Symptoms		IP with Symptoms	
1.	GI	.3763**	GI	.4251**	GI	.2960**
2.	GAD	.3193**	GAD	.3481**	GAD	.3320**
3.	REPR	.1734**	REPR	.3356**	REPR	.1902**
4.	NM	.2250	NM	.3615**	NM	.3395**
5.	SKIN	.2413**	SKIN	.3267**	SKIN	.3056**
6.	CVR	.3216**	CVR	.3279**	CVR	.2849**

**P .01
*P .05

1. If a woman was in the second or third trimester, her first trimester symptoms were based on recollection. If she was in her third trimester then the second and first trimester symptoms were based upon recollection.

We totaled the score of all the stress scales and called the index STRESS. Similarly, we totaled all the scores of the pregnancy symptom scales and called that index TOTAL.

References

Engel. G.L. & Schmale, A.H., Jr. (1965 April). The psychological setting of somatic illness. Paper presented before the American College of Physicians, New York, N.Y.; quoted by Thurlow.

Hinkle, L.E., Jr. (1959). Physical health, mental health and the social environment: some characteristics of healthy and unhealthy people. In recent contributions of biological and psychosocial investigations to preventive psychiatry. In R.H. Ojemann (Ed.), *Proceedings of the 2nd Institute of Preventive Psychiatry,* Iowa State University Press, Ames, Iowa (p. 79).

Holmes, T.S. & Holmes, T.H. (1970). Short-term intrusions into the lifestyle routine. *Journal of Psychosomatic Research, 14,* 121.

Holmes. T.H. & Rahe, R.H. (1967). The social readjustment rating scale. *Journal of Psychosomatic Research, 11,* 213.

Rahe, R.H. (1969). Multi-Cultural correlation of life change scaling: America, Japan, Denmark, and Sweden. *Journal of Psychosomatic Research, 13,* 191.

Rahe, R.H. (1969). Life crisis and health change. In P.R.A. May & J.R. Wittenborn (Eds.), *Psychotropic drug response: Advances in prediction* (p. 92). Springfield: C.C. Thomas.

Rahe, R.H. & Arthur, R.J. (1968). Life change patterns surrounding illness experience. *Journal of Psychosomatic Research, 11,* 341.

Rahe, R.H., Gunderson, E.K.E., & Arthur R.J. (1970). Demographic and psychosocial factors in acute illness reporting. *Journal of Chronic Diseases, 23,* 245.

Rahe, R.H., Lundberg, U., Bennett, L., & Theorell, T. (1971). The social readjustment rating scale: A comparative study of Swedes and Americans. *Journal of Psychosomatic Research, 15,* 241.

Rahe, R.H., Mahan, J., & Arthur, R.J. (1970). Prediction of near-future health change from subjects' preceding life changes. *Journal of Psychosomatic Research, 14,* 401.

Rahe, R.H. (1972). Subjects' recent life changes and their near-future illness reports. *Annals of Clinical Research, 4,* 250-265.

Thurlow, H.J. (1967). General susceptibility to illness: A selective review. *Canadian Medical Association Journal, 97,* 1397-1404.

Selected Bibliography

Abramson, J.H., Singh, A.R., & Mbambo, V. (1961). Antenatal stress and the baby's development. *Archives of Disease in Childhood, 36,* 42-49.

Aubry, R.H. & Nesbitt, R.E.L. (1969). High-risk obstetrics. *American Journal of Obstetrics and Gynecology, 105,* 2, 241-247.

Babson, S.G. & Denson, R.C. (1971). *Management of high-risk pregnancy and intensive care of the neonate.* St. Louis: Mosby.

Beck, J.C. & Worthen, K. (1972). Precipitating stress, crisis theory, and hospitalization in schizophrenia and depression. *Archives of General Psychiatry, 26,* 123-129.

Blau, A., Slaff, B., Easton, K., Welkowitz, J., Springarn, J., & Cohen, J. (1963). The psychogenic etiology of premature births. *Psychosomatic Medicine, 25,* 3, 201-211.

Burstein, I., Kinch, R.A.H., & Stern, L. (1974). Anxiety, pregnancy, labor and the neonate. *American Journal of Obstretics and Gynecology, 118,* 2, 195-199.

Butler, N.R. (1963). *Perinatal mortality: The first report of the 1958 British prenatal mortality survey.* Edinburgh: E. & S. Livingstone, Ltd.

Butler, N.R. & Alberman, E.D. (Eds.) (1969). *Perinatal problems: The second report of the 1958 British perinatal mortality survey.* Edinburgh: E. & S. Livingstone.

Cline, D.W. & Chosy, J.J. (1972). A prospective study of life changes and subsequent health changes. *Archives of General Psychiatry, 27,* 51-53.

Coddington, R.D. (1971). The significance of life events as etiological factors in the diseases of children. *Journal of Psychosomatic Research, 16,* 7-18.

Coddington, R.D. (1972). The significance of life events as etiological factors in the diseases of children — II. A study of a normal population. *Journal of Psychosomatic Research, 16,* 205-213.

Cohen, J. (1969). *Statistical power analysis for the behavioral sciences.* New York: Academic Press.

Cook, T.D. & Campbell, D.T. (1979). *Quasi-experimentation: Design and analysis issues for field settings.* Chicago: Rand McNally.

Coppen, A.J. (1958). Psychosomatic aspects of pre-eclampic toxemia. *Journal of Psychosomatic Research, 2,* 241-265.

Davids, A. & DeVault, S. (1962). Maternal anxiety during pregnancy and childbirth abnormalities. *Psychosomatic Medicine, 24,* 5, 464-470.

Davids, A. & Rosengren, W.R. (1962). Social stability and psychological adjustment during pregnancy. *Psychosomatic Medicine, 24,* 6, 579-583.

Dohrenwend, B.S. (1973). Life events as stressors: A methodological inquiry. *Journal of Health & Social Behavior, 14,* 2, 167-175.

Downs, F. (1964). Maternal stress in primigravidas as a factor in the production of neonatal pathology. *Nursing Science, 2,* 348-367.

Friederich, M.A., Romano, J., & Lund, C.J. (1963). Psychologic aspects of obstetric-gynecologic practice. *American Journal of Obstetrics and Gynecology,* 1029-1033.

Grimm, E.R. (1961). Psychological tension in pregnancy. *Psychosomatic Medicine, 23,* 6, 520-527.

Gunter, L.M. (1963). Psychopathology and stress in the life experience of mothers of premature infants. *American Journal of Obstetrics and Gynecology, 86,* 3, 333-340.

Hawkins, N.G., Davis, R., & Holmes, T.H. (1957). Evidence of psychosocial factors in the development of pulmonary tuberculosis. *American Review of Tuberculosis and Pulmonary Diseases, 75,* 5.

Hetzel, B.S., Bruer, B., & Poidevin, L.O.S. (1961). A survey of the relation between certain common antenatal complications in primiparae and stressful life situations during pregnancy. *Journal of Psychosomatic Research, 5,* 175-182.

Knoblock, H. & Pasamanick, B. (1960). Environmental factors affecting human development before and after birth. *Pediatrics,* 210-218.

Komaroff, A.L., Masuda, M., & Holmes, T.H. (1968). The social readjustment rating scale: A comparative study of Negro, Mexican, and White Americans. *Journal of Psychosomatic Research, 12,* 121.

Korones, S.B. (1972). *High risk newborn infants: The basis for intensive nursing care.* St. Louis: Mosby.

Kuhn, T.S. (1962). *The structure of scientific revolutions.* Chicago: University of Chicago Press.

Lewis, R., Charles, M., & Patwary, K.M. (1973). Relationships between birth weight and selected social, environmental, and medical care factors. *American Journal of Public Health, 63,* 11, 973-981.

Masuda, A.Z. & Holmes, T.H. (1967). The social readjustment rating scale: A cross-cultural study of Japanese and Americans. *Journal of Psychsomatic Research, 11,* 227.

McDonald, R.L. (1968). The role of emotional factors in obstetric complications: A review. *Psychosomatic Medicine, 30,* 222-237.

McDonald, R.L., Gynther, M.D., & Christakos, A.C. (1963). Relations between maternal anxiety and obstetric complications. *Psychosomatic Medicine, 25,* 4, 357-353.

Myers, J.K., Lindenthal, J.J., Pepper, M.P., & Ostrander, D.R. (1972). Life events and mental status: A longitudinal study. *Journal of Health and Social Behavior, 13,* 398-406.

Myrianthopoulas, N.C. & French, K.S. (1968). An application of the U.S. bureau of the census socioeconomic index to a large, diversified patient population. *Social Science & Medicine, 2,* 283-299.

Nam, C.B. & Powers, M.G. (1965). Variations in socioeconomic structure by race, residence and the life cycle. *American Sociological Review, 30,* 97.

Niswander, K.R. & Gordon, M. (Eds.) (1972). *The women and their pregnancies.* Collaborative Perinatal Study of the National Institute of Neurological Disease and Stroke. Philadelphia: Saunders.

Nuckolls, K.B., Cassel, J., & Kaplan, B.H. (1972). Psychosocial assets, life crisis and the prognosis of pregnancy. *American Journal of Epidemiology, 95,* 5, 431-441.

Paykel, E.S., Prusoff, B.A., Uhlenhuth, E.H. (1971). Scaling of life events. *Archives of General Psychiatry, 25,* 340-347.

Pedhazur, E.J. (1982). *Multiple regression in behavioral research* (2nd ed.), (p. 582). New York: Holt, Rinehart and Winston.

Rahe, R.H. (1969). Life crisis and health change. In P.R.A. May 8. J.R. Wittenborn (Eds.), *Psychotropic drug response: Advances in prediction* (p. 92). Springfield: C.C. Thomas.

Roghmann, K.J. & Haggerty, R.J. (1973). Daily stress, illness, and use of health services in young families. *Pediatric Research, 7,* 520-526.

Satin, D.G. (1972). (Help): Life stresses and psycho-social problems in the hospital emergency unit. *Social Psychiatry, 7,* 119-126.

Schaie, K.W. (1965). A general model for the study of developmental problems. *Psychological Bulletin, 64,* 2, 92-107.

Smith, A.C., Flick, G.L., Ferriss, G.S., & Sellmann, A.H. (1972). Prediction of developmental outcome at seven years from prenatal, perinatal, and postnatal events. *Child Development, 43,* 495-507.

Smith, W.G. (1971). Critical life-events and prevention strategies in mental health. *Archives of General Psychiatry, 25,* 102-109.

Stott, D.H. (1958). Some psychosomatic aspects of casualty in reproduction. *Journal of Psychosomatic Research, 3,* 42-55.

Stott, D.H. (1974). Follow-up study from birth on the effects of prenatal stress. *Developmental Medicine and Child Neurology, 118,* 2, 195-199.

Thomson, K.C. & Nedrie, H.C. (1972). Environmental stress in primary depressive illness. *Archives of General Psychiatry, 26,* 130-132.

Thurlow, H.J. (1971). Illness in relation to life situation and sick role tendency. *Journal of Psychosomatic Research, 15,* 73.

Uhlenhuth, E.H. & Paykel, E.S. (1973). Symptom intensity and life events. *Archives of General Psychiatry, 28,* 473-477.

2

Two Studies Of The Pregnancy Process

We have described the evolution of our theories and the development of our PIPAS scales. Although there have been some interesting minor research studies (appendices B, C, D), we are now in a position to use the system of variables to see how they describe the process of pregnancy.

The original hypotheses came from (a) clinical observations and general presuppositions of practitioners, (b) reflections on the research literature on stress and pregnancy, and (c) general conceptions of a philosophy of science. Inasmuch as we have discussed the first two sources previously, we will only comment briefly on the third component.

As is well known, most scientists spend their professional lives doing what Kuhn (1962) calls "normal science." These activities are primarily the gradual development of a set of assumptions by the scientific community. By slow accretion, knowledge accumulates, frequently by a dialetical process of experiment and counter-experiment.

Most theoretical conceptions involve only a partial set of variables, that is, they are incomplete. Because of this incompleteness anomalies develop. In an effort to account for these anomalies the problems are re-conceptualized. When this happens on a fundamental level in science, we have scientific revolutions. On small scale scientific problems like the PIPAS Project we either abandon, change, or enlarge the theoretical apparatus. In our case we initially enlarged the "Stress leads to illness" paradigm to "stress and symptom proness influence pregnancy symptoms" directly and indirectly through a personality variable Cornell Psychiatric Items, (CPI).

At this point of our research program we decide to make a break from the traditional studies and take seriously the talk about "process" as in "the pregnancy process." Process laws require fairly strict conditions: (a) a system with strong bounderies; (b) a system in which all the variables and their relationships are known; and (c) a system whose state at one time is known.

The process law allows the prediction of successive states of a system. The classic example is the planetary system. The lack of a true process law results frequently in a primitive approximation of narrow "stages." The division of pregnancy into "trimesters" roughly corresponds to "stages." The temporal regularity of pregnancy makes the division into trimesters cogent.

The technical development in statistics and measurement of path analyses made possible an attempt to construct a partial process description of pregnancy. We had developed some of the necessary measures, had the path-analytic methodology, had the cooperation of many pregnant women, and also had the insight into the scientific advantages of attempting even a partial process description. The following are the results of the combination of these factors.

Procedure

Consent.

All subjects participating in this research were given on the first page of the survey form standard information on the risks, benefits, and guarantees of anonymity of participating in the research (see Appendix A). In addition, they were asked for permission to review their hospital labor and delivery medical records.

Sample

There were 1330 pregnant primigravid women in this study. We selected primigravid women so that responses to pregnancy would not be influenced by previous pregnancy experiences. This sample of women constitutes part of the 2404 pregnant women of the PIPAS Project Data Base. These women were sets of convenience samples collected from seven hospitals distributged throughout Utah with a maximum concentration in the Salt Lake valley. There was one sample of 300 women from an inner-city hospital in Phoenix, Arizona. The women were participating in prenatal classes or attending prenatal clinics. Many of the women who live crisis life-styles, who have low socioeconomic-educational levels, and who are members of ethnic subgroups are not represented in this data base with the same distributions as they appear in the general population. The women in the data base, however, are a fair sample of women who attend prenatal classes and clinics in the Intermountain West. Their demographic characterists are given in Table 1.

Measures

The Symptom-Proneness Scale is described in Chapter 1. A list of these items is in Table 8 of that chapter. The Alpha coefficient of this scale is .80, based upon 1330 primigravidas.

The STRESS measures were constructed for each month of pregnancy by taking the total number of symptoms women reported (TOTAL) and regressing this variable on the total score of the Utah Stress Scales. The resulting regression equation provided the weights for the individual scales for the construction of the STRESS variable. The individual stress scales are short versions of those discussed in Chapter 1, the items of which can be seen in Appendix A. The Alpha coefficients are based upon 1330 primigravidas.

Scale	Alpha Coefficient
Family Stress	.62
Lifestyle Stress	.61
Personal Habit Change Stress	.77
Work Stress	.83
Social Stress	.67
Financial Stress	.61

TABLE 1

Demographic Data on Subjects for Path Analyses, June 1978
1330 Primagravidas*

Ages of Pregnant Women

Mean	21.939
Standard Deviation	3.404
Minimum	13
Maximum	40
Missing Values	9
Valid Cases	1321

Educational Level

0-6 Grade	1
7-9 Grade	17
10-11 Grade	92
High School Graduate	458
At Least One Year College	441
College Graduate	159
Post College Graduate	43
Mising Values	119
Valid Cases	1211

Marital Status

Single	65
Married	1242
Widowed/Divorced/Separated	15
Missing Values	8
Valid Cases	1322

Number of Months Pregnant at Time of Taking Utah

2	8
3	53
4	104
5	166
6	281
7	378
8	256
9	68
10	1
Missing Values	15
Valid Cases	1315

Was Pregnancy Planned?

No	460
Yes	811
Missing Values	59
Valid Cases	1271

* These data are based on women from both Utah and Arizona who planned to deliver in nine different hospitals.

The final criterion, endogenous variable, the total number of symptoms women reported, was simply the total symptoms from the set of six symptom scales: Gastrointestinal, General Adaptational Distress, Reproductive, Neuromuscular, skin, and Cardiovascular-Respiratory, symptoms. Based upon 1330 primigravidas, the total set of symptoms in the first trimester had an Alpha coefficient of .71, in the second trimester an Alpha coefficient of .82, and in the third trimester an Alpha coefficient of .93.

Statistical Analyses

All the path coefficients were obtained from the beta weights of regression equations when the CPA was regressed on STRESS and the CPI, and when TOTAL was regressed on the set STRESS, SP, and CPI. These path coefficients are, therefore, standardized partial regression coefficients. These coefficients indicate the magnitude of change in standard deviation units that one could expect in the effect variable with a one-unit change in the causal variable. This change represents the unique contribution of the causal variable, independent of the other causal variables. The Statistical Package for the Social Sciences (SPSS) regression procedure was used for all these analyses.

Results and Discussion

The present study is cross-sectional rather than longitudinal. This design has strengths and weaknesses, as do all designs (Schaie, 1965). Inferences from data in the present study depend on the equivalency of the various groups of women in the different months of pregnancy. A longitudinal design would have avoided this problem since the same women would have been tested each month; however, it would have been more difficult on the participants. Whereas a longitudinal design would have eliminated the potential problem of sampling variations in each group, it would have created problems of its own, such as possible reactivity due to repeated measurements (Cook and Campbell, 1979) or attrition. Indeed, Schaie has suggested that longitudinal studies are basically inefficient. A longitudinal design was used for the Childbearing Year data reported in Chapter 3, with the resultant expected attrition reducing the size of the third trimester data set.

In addition, Pedhazur (1982, p. 582) notes tht one of the assumptions of causal analyses is that each residual is not correlated with the variables which precede it in a model. Thus the residuals for month five, for instance, should not be correlated with variables of months six, seven, eight or nine. The same general prescription applies to successive testing of persons in longitudinal studies. In this study the women in each month of pregnancy are a different set.

Inferences drawn about the course of pregnancy based on the present design depend on the assumption that the women in each month of pregnancy are equivalent, or, more accurately, that the women were equivalent prior to the pregnancy. This latter distinction is important because the intent of this research is to investigate differences among the women related to the month of pregnancy. Two measures collected were "historical," those having to do with life changes 6-12 months ago (STRESS 2), and with symptoms experienced during the last 10 years (SP). Testing to see if the groups of women were significantly different on these measures provided a check of the assumption of group equivalency. Two ANOVA's were conducted. Differences among the groups were not significant — STRESS 2:F=2.544, df (6,1299), p=05. SP:F=1.580, df=, (6,1299), p=05.

Women in the different months of pregnancy seem to have had an equivalent or similar number of symptoms during the past 10 years (score on SP) and an equivalent number of life changes 6-12 months ago (STRESS 2). However, changes occuring 0-6 months ago (STRESS) are more predictive of TOTAL symptoms during pregnancy and so this measure was used in the path analyses. The women were significantly different in the number of life changes 0-6 months ago which suggests that each month of pregnancy has a different typical number of life changes (STRESS: F=2.544, df (6.1299), p .05). And, in fact, inspection of the mean number of life changes for women in each successive month of pregnancy shows an increasingly greater number, with one small exception in the fourth month (see Table 2).

Relations of Stress to Symptom Proneness (SP)

The results of this work are displayed in Figures 1 to 6. The conventional interpretation is given to the path diagrams. Connecting

STRESS and SYMPTOM PRONENESS is an arcing line with no arrows. These are exogenous variables, the index number of which is the correlation between the two variables. These correlations average r=.30, thus 9% of the variance is common to both variables.

We think of women as not only symptom-prone but also as stress-prone. Thus, there is some presumption that those who are stress-prone tend also to be symptom-prone. This relationship at the conceptual level, however, is not reflected in item overlaps, for the stress items are largely life situations (have a mortgage, graduated from school, gotten married, etc.) during the last six months or year. The symptom items are such things as headaches or stiff joints that a woman has had over the last ten years of her life.

Relations of the Stress and Symptom Proneness (SP) to Cornell Psychiatric Items (CPI)

An inspection of the CPI items in Table 9 of Chapter 1 indicates that these are fairly extreme emotional conditions. If a person responds positively to more than three of these items the general interpretation is that they ought to be carefully observed to see if they need some sort of psychological help. It is of interest that the path coefficients of the CPI, STRESS are consistently higher than those of CPI, SP. This makes sense to us because physical symptoms are quite a distinct domain from the psychological items. As a result of these path analyses we now think it would be easy to construct a "psychological symptom proneness scale" that would include items like sleep difficulties, constant worry, etc. over the last ten years.

As far as the general course of pregnancy, it can be seen that the fifth month has the highest CPI score, and that in terms of prediction the multiple correlation was highest (R=.72187) on the ninth month. The CPI, STRESS path coefficient was highest in the eighth month. An inspection of the path coefficients for the eighth and ninth months reveals an interesting dynamic about how stress works in late pregnancy. Notice the path coefficient CPI, STRESS8 is .42649 while the path coefficient TOTAL8, STRESS8 is only .16763. This means, of course, that the major effect of stress on total symptoms is through the effect of stress on CPI, and then on total symptoms. The contrast in the next month is

TABLE 2
Means by Month (SD)

Measure	Month 3	4	5	6	7	8	9
CPI	2.40 (3.02)	2.29 (3.26)	3.06 (3.30)	2.90 (3.54)	2.05 (3.26)	3.00 (3.38)	2.35 (2.29)
SP	5.58 (3.91)	6.21 (4.09)	6.34 (3.74)	5.79 (3.79)	5.58 (3.84)	5.54 (3.95)	5.13 (3.93)
STRESS	11.04 (7.98)	10.85 (7.55)	11.49 (7.24)	11.78 (6.89)	12.78 (7.12)	12.94 (6.93)	13.54 (7.65)
STRESS 2	5.53 (6.39)	4.75 (4.81)	5.27 (5.08)	5.36 (5.45)	5.38 (4.95)	6.34 (6.06)	5.46 (5.03)
CASES	53	104	166	281	378	256	68

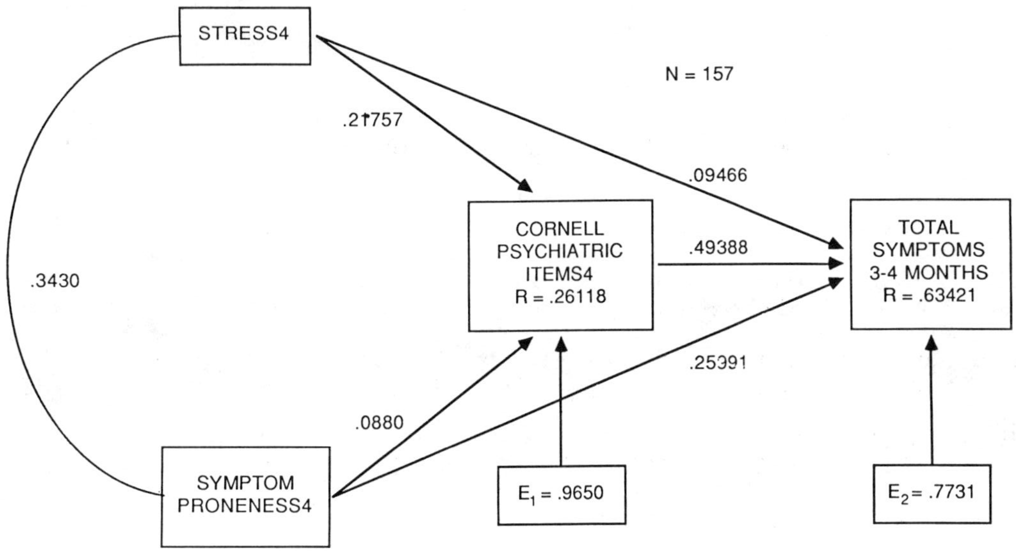

	MEAN	SD	CORRELATIONS TOTAL4	CPI4	SP4	STRESS4
TOTAL4	12.293	6.070	1.0000	.5596	.3727	.3061
CPI4	1.841	2.340		1.0000	.1626	.2478
SP4	6.000	4.032			1.0000	.3430
STRESS4	12.215	1.828				1.0000

FIGURE 1. Relations of Stress Index, Symptom Proneness Index, Cornell Psychiatric Items to Total Symptoms Reported By Primagravidas Who Were 3-4 Months Pregnant, 1978.

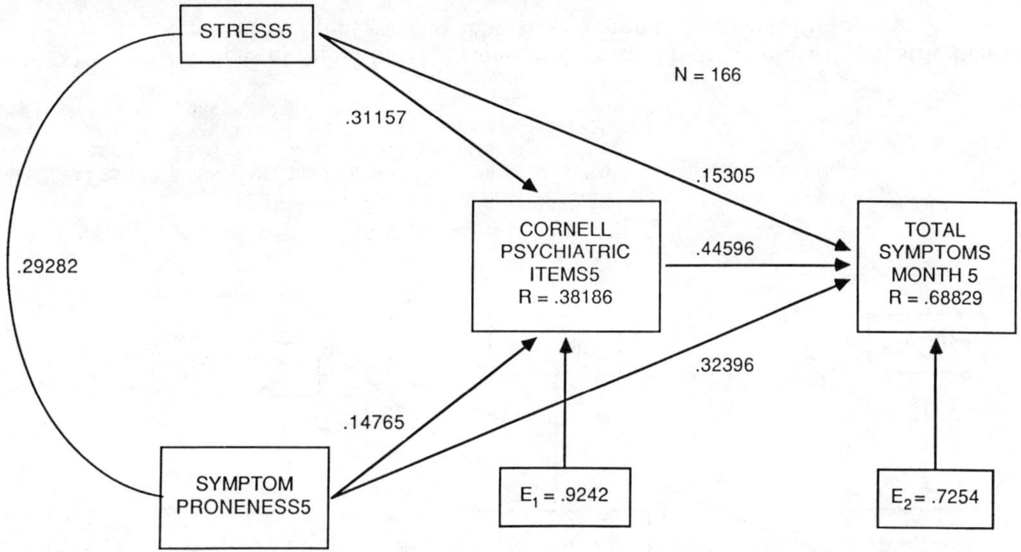

	MEAN	SD	CORRELATIONS TOTAL5	CPI5	SP5	STRESS5
TOTAL5	14.596	7.161	1.0000	.5777	.4753	.4061
CPI5	3.060	3.304		1.0000	.2388	.3548
SP5	6.337	3.744			1.0000	.2928
STRESS5	14.598	2.908				1.0000

FIGURE 2. Relations of Stress Index, Symptom Proneness Index, Cornell Psychiatric Items to Total Symptoms Reported By Primagravidas Who Were 5 Months Pregnant, 1978.

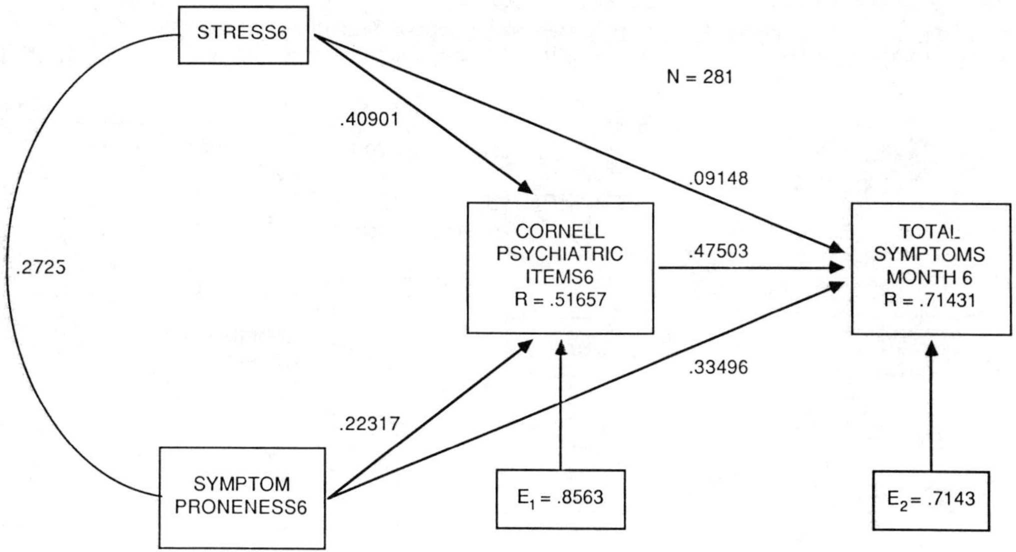

	MEAN	SD	TOTAL6	CPI6	SP6	STRESS6
			CORRELATIONS			
TOTAL6	14.214	6.896	1.0000	.6301	.5189	.4060
CPI6	2.900	3.535		1.0000	.3346	.4698
SP6	5.787	3.786			1.0000	.2725
STRESS6	14.828	3.085				1.0000

FIGURE 3. Relations of Stress Index, Symptom Proneness Index, Cornell Psychiatric Items to Total Symptoms Reported By Primagravidas Who Were 6 Months Pregnant, 1978.

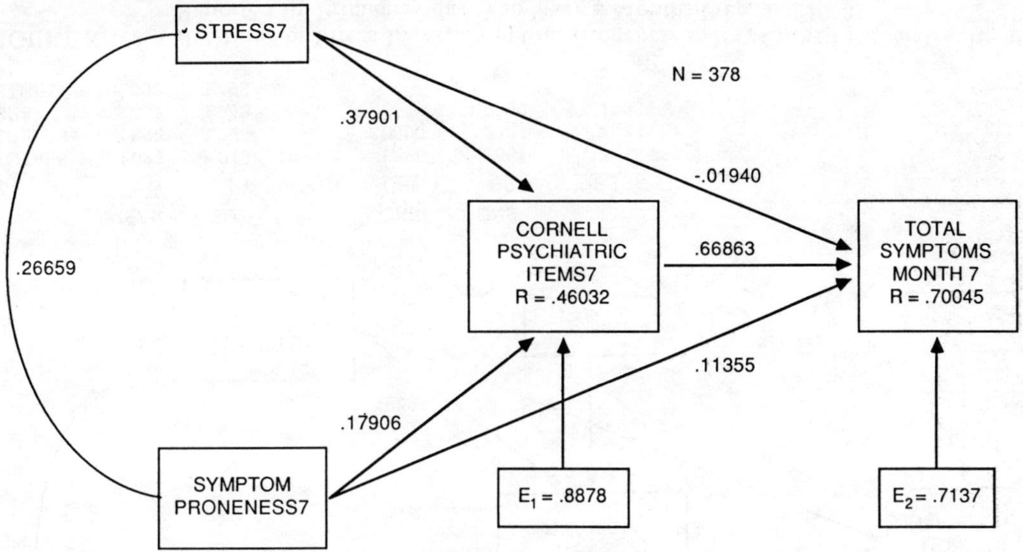

	MEAN	SD	TOTAL7	CPI7	SP7	STRESS7
			CORRELATIONS			
TOTAL7	10.571	8.821	1.0000	.6922	.2957	.2962
CPI7	2.048	3.264		1.0000	.2801	.4268
SP7	5.582	3.840			1.0000	.2666
STRESS7	10.571	2.613				1.0000

FIGURE 4. Relations of Stress Index, Symptom Proneness Index, Cornell Psychiatric Items to Total Symptoms Reported By Primagravidas Who Were 7 Months Pregnant, 1978.

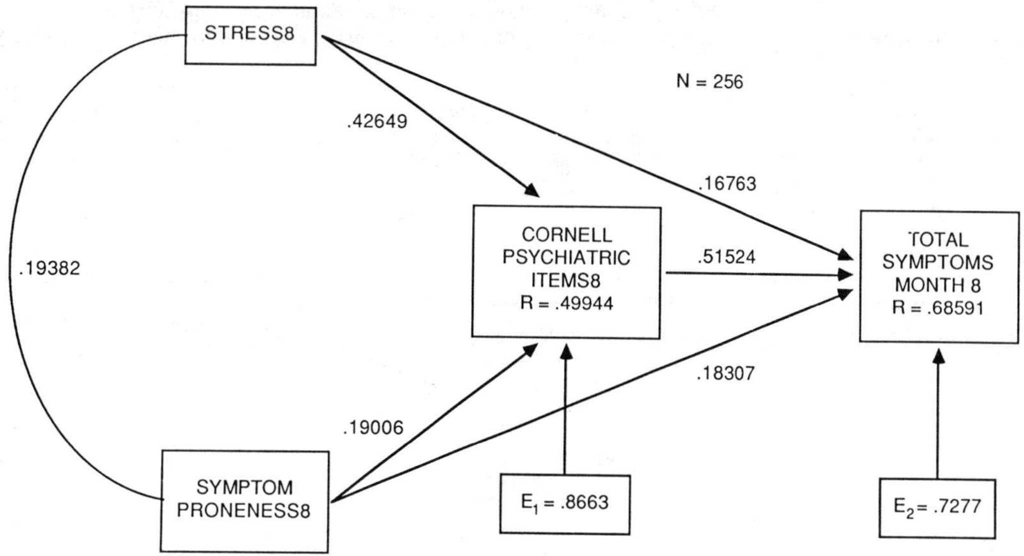

	MEAN	SD	CORRELATIONS TOTAL8	CPI8	SP8	STRESS8
TOTAL8	16.098	7.919	1.0000	.6428	.3561	.4418
CPI8	2.996	3.374		1.0000	.2727	.4633
SP8	5.438	3.948			1.0000	.1938
STRESS8	16.098	3.499				1.0000

FIGURE 5. Relations of Stress Index, Symptom Proneness Index, Cornell Psychiatric Items to Total Symptoms Reported By Primagravidas Who Were 8 Months Pregnant, 1978.

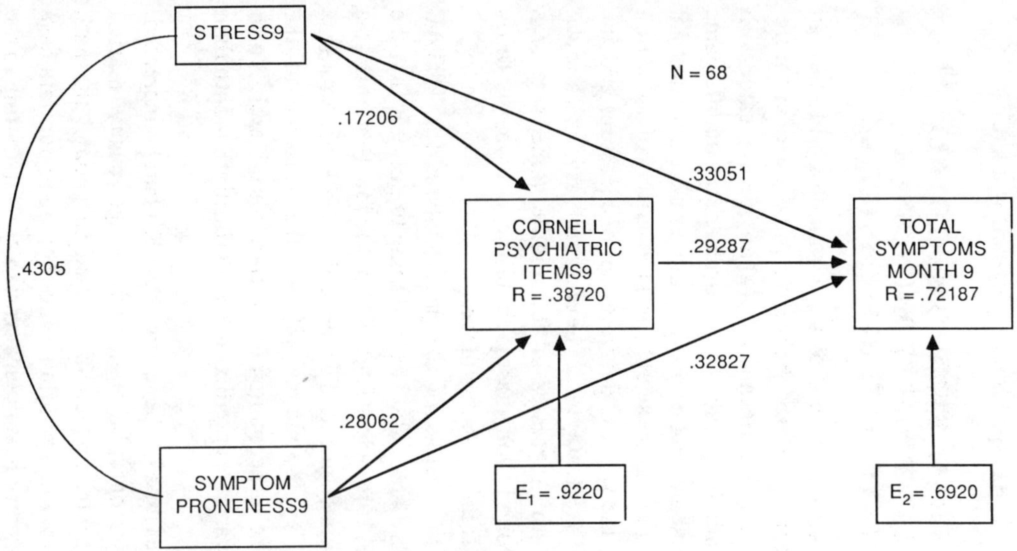

	MEAN	SD	CORRELATIONS TOTAL9	CPI9	SP9	STRESS9
TOTAL9	17.294	7.583	1.0000	.5061	.5745	.5576
CPI9	2.353	2.291		1.0000	.3547	.2928
SP9	5.132	3.928			1.0000	.4305
STRESS9	17.285	3.928				1.0000

FIGURE 6. Relations of Stress Index, Symptom Proneness Index, Cornell Psychiatric Items to Total Symptoms Reported By Primagravidas Who Were 9 Months Pregnant, 1978.

striking. CPI, STRESS9 is reduced to .17206 while TOTAL9, STRESS9 is increased to .33051. The effect of stress in the eighth month is on psychological states, but the effect in the ninth month is on physical states. Our general prescription is that the eighth month is a difficult period of pregnancy psychologically and that stresses during these months should be carefully managed by the pregnant women.

Relations of TOTAL SYMPTOMS (TOTAL) to STRESS, SYMPTOM PRONENESS (SP), CORNELL PSYCHIATRIC ITEMS (CPI).

In philosophy there is frequent use of the terminology of chess in discussions, perhaps because much of the work has a dialectical nature. This research, however, can be patterned into (a) an opening game with opening moves, (b) a middle game with characteristic middle-game moves, and (c) and an end game. The opening moves were a theoretical analysis of the problem, a literature search, and the writing of a research proposal. The middle game was the development of measures and the collection of the large PIPAS Data Base. The end game, as is well known, is really determined by the successes of the middle game, sort of a consolidation of the ground won inasmuch as the outcome is fairly predictable. This report is an end-game move.

Figures 1 to 6 give the results of the path analyses for TOTAL symptoms to STRESS, SP and CPI. The first thing to notice is that the multiple correlation goes from a low R=.63421 in the fourth month to a high of R=.72187 in the ninth month. The mean R is .69084; its square is .4773. On an average, approximately 48% of the variance of the pregnancy symptoms is being accounted for by these variables. It is also clear that our system of variables predicts better in the ninth month than in the fourth month.

There are two good reasons for believing these R's can be increased. First, there are much demographic data such as age, parity, marital status, educational level, etc. that could be used to expand the path diagrams. There is, however, a limitation of not having in our data base measures of good concurrent physiological variables contributing to the prediction of pregnancy symptoms. Second, the data tend to be positively skewed, as data on proneness tend to be. Thus the linear assumptions do not fit closely the actual data. If the data are split into below the mean and above the mean on TOTAL, then the below-half regression equations R's tend to be markedly lower than those of the upper half. Although in terms of elegant simplicity this is not good (violates linear models assumption mildly), clinically it is of great interest that our measures increase their precision of description at the high end of the continuum of symptoms where there is a natural concentration of clinical attention.

Most surprising of all the findings were the dynamic changes between the path coefficients from the seventh month on. In this month the path coefficient TOTAL, CPI = .6683 while the contributions of SP and STRESS are .11355 and -.0194, respectively. In the ninth month there is a rise in both STRESS and SP along with a drop in the contribution of CPI. The change is so dramatic that it is believed to be real.

Given any set of data, the experienced and conceptually agile clinician can think of a possible explanation. Whereas the explanation is *ex post facto,* and, logically, many premises may be constructed to explain a conclusion, the explanations are not worth much. With these caveats in mind, the following hypothesis is offered: as the physiological load of pregnancy increases past the seventh month, the adaptive physiological and psychological range or adaptive reserve (coping resources) decreases. Thus the additional load of stress and symptom vulnerability will be detectable in the rise of the path coefficients. The drop in the path coefficient TOTAL, CPI during the last month is so dramatic that it might well be a reflection of a physiological variable, like the secretion of the ovarian hormone relaxin, which reaches its peak about the 38th to 40th week. We suggest that its psychological analogue is to reduce the hugely pregnant woman into a passive waiting state in which there is a muting of emotional reactions. But more research on this hypothesis is needed.

At best, the results of our path analysis show the importance of symptom proneness and personality to stress in predicting pregnancy symptoms. Yet the multiple regression levels show that we are far from knowing all the relevant variables of the pregnancy system. We now know, as a result of subsequent research, that we can push our regression equations to account for 70% of variance of symptoms by the addition of nutritional and aerobic variables.

The limits of how far we can go are probably determined by physiological variables. What has amazed us is how much of the minor symptoms, which make pregnancy such a trial, are attributed to social, environmental, and crude internal factors such as symptom proneness and a crude measure of psychological distress.

Study of High Stress, High Symptom Proneness, etc.:

The second series of studies are tests of our original hypothesis that both symptom proneness and stress affect the course and quality of the pregnancy. There were two problems in the testing of this hypothesis. The first was to select a dependent variable whose natural occurrence in pregnancy was high and quite variable among women. Obviously a variable that was low in occurrence or one that had little variability among women would be unlikely to be sensitively related to stress and symptom proneness.

Put in another way, one could say having selected minor pregnancy symptoms as a criterion variable, the research problem was to determine its relation to symptom proneness and stress. The minor pregnancy symptoms, the criterion variable, was the total number of symptoms of the various symptom scales, Gastrointestinal, General Adaptational Distress, Reproductive, Neuromuscular, Skin, and Cardiovascular-Respiratory, as listed in Appendix A. The independent variables were High and Low Stress, and High and Low Symptom Proneness. To determine the exact limits of these variables, the following procedure was used. The six-month pregnant women were arbitrarily selected, and frequencies were computed for total stress measures (total of work, financial, family, personal habit changes, life-style, and social stress scales.) As near as possible the upper and lower 20% of pregnant women on these scales were selected. The exact parameters were:

High Symptom Proneness, High Stress	SP=7, Stress=17
High Symptom Proneness, Low Stress	SP=7, Stress=7
Low Symptom Proneness, High Stress	SP=3, Stress=17
Low Symptom Proneness, Low Stress	SP=3, Stress=7

Thus, for instance, in each trimester the high symptom proneness combined with the high stress group were women who reported greater than 7 symptoms and also checked greater than 17 stresses. Similarly, the low symptom proneness and low stress group reported less than 3 symptoms and also less than 7 stresses.

Our hypotheses and our predictions were that highly stressed and symptom prone women would report many more pregnancy symptoms than those women who were not highly stressed and not symptom prone. The results are in Table 3 and Figure 7.

Our hypotheses were confirmed beyond our expectation. And we are provided a lesson in the differences between clinical and theoretical conjectures, and (the results of) empirical research. The conjecture that stressed people would report more pregnancy symptoms than non-stressed individuals was not difficult to formulate. Similarly the conjecture that symptom-prone individuals would report more symptoms than symptom-resistant individuals was also not difficult to formulate.

If we distinguish four levels of linguistic precision roughly corresponding to levels of measurement, (a) nominal, (b) ordinal, (c) interval and (d) ratio, the clinical and theoretical hypotheses of this research program were at the semi-quantitative or ordinal level. One group of women will have more symptoms than another group. In this research the problem was not merely the ordinal relationship but how many symptoms would each group report. At this point the clinical and our present theoretical formulations were of no help.

Only empirical research provides answers to the question of how large were the differences between the High Stress and High Symptom-Prone group and the group with Low Stress and Low Symptom Proneness. In general, the high group had almost three times the number of pregnancy symptoms of the low group. As an aside, we mention that the low group, who report on an average seven pregnancy symptoms for each trimester, represent an ideal goal. This is, through management of stress, and general health of pregnant women, particularly in the pre-pregnancy period, we would like to transform the high stress and high symptom-prone groups to report the pregnancy symptoms of the lowest group.

It is apparent that in the third trimester, compared with the first and second trimester, the role of stress is enhanced. Comparing the first two

TABLE 3

Total Number of Pregnancy Symptom for Each Trimester of Each Four Groups

GROUP	CONDITION	TRIMESTER I.	II.	III.
I.	High Symptom Proneness High Stress	18.667	19.735	20.141
II.	High Symptom Proneness Low Stress	13.750	16.273	11.762
III.	Low Symptom Proneness High Stress	7.500	10.000	14.629
IV.	Low Symptom Proneness Low Stress	7.200	6.484	7.883

groups, it is apparent that during the third trimester low stress markedly reduced the number of pregnancy symptoms reported. Conversely, high stress in the low symptom-prone group markedly increased the number of reported pregnancy symptoms. The path analyses confirm the general trend with the further speciication that the effect of the stress variables is largest in the ninth month.

These striking findings are important for nursing and medical caregivers. The recommendation is to reduce stress factors as much as possible in the third trimester and particularly in the ninth month.

It is also of interest that the first three groups show a progression in reported symptoms from the first through the third trimester. By contrast, the fourth group shows a drop in reported symptoms in the second trimester.

Chapter 3 details how these scales and research finding were applied in a comprehensive program of prenatal education. The response of clincians and expectant couples is described.

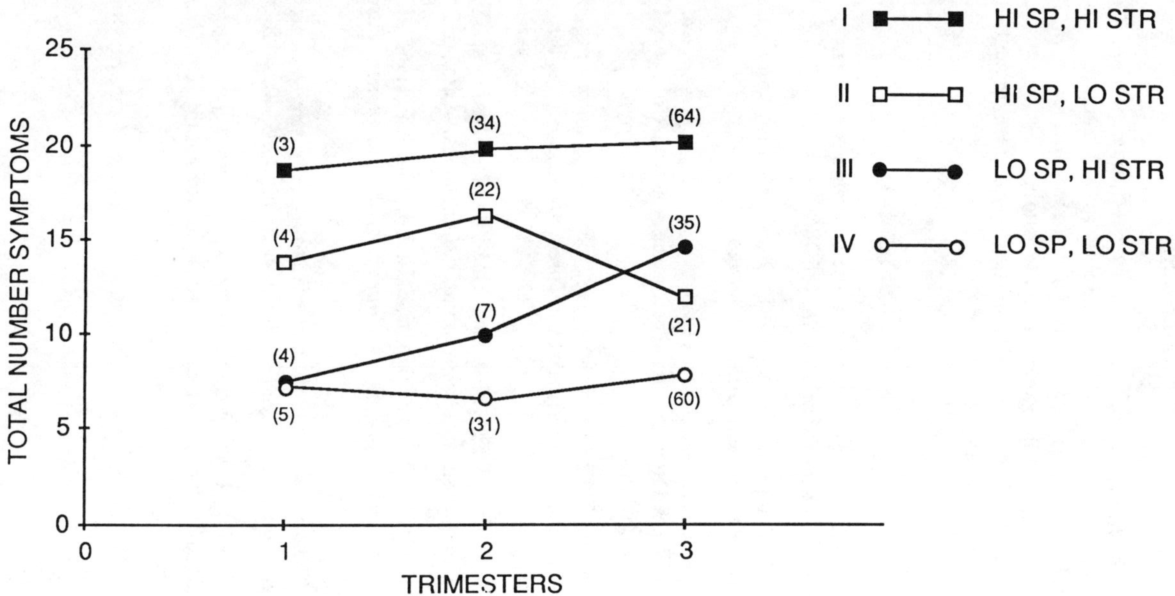

FIGURE 7. Reported Pregnancy Symptoms of High and Low Symptom Proneness and Stress Groups.

References

Cook, T.D. & Campbell, D.T. (1979). *Quasi-experimentation: Design and analysis issues for field settings.* Chicago: Rand McNally.

Pedhazur, E.J. (1982). *Multiple regression in behavioral research* (2nd ed., p. 582). New York: Holt, Rinehart and Winston.

Schaie, K.W. (1965). A general model for the study of developmental problems. *Psychological Bulletin, 64,* 2, 92-107.

Selected Bibliography

Coddington, R.D. (1979). Life events associated with adolescent pregnancies. *Journal of Clinical Psychiatry, 40,* 180-185.

Cook, T.D. & Campbell, D.T. (1979). *Quasi-experimentation: Design and analysis issues for field settings.* Chicago: Rand McNally.

Engel, G.L. & Schmale, A.H., Jr. (1965, April). *The psychological setting of somatic illness.* Paper presented before the American College of Physicians, New York, N.Y.

Fagley, N., Miller, P., & Sullivan J. (1982). Stress, symptom proneness, and general adaptational distress during pregnancy. *Journal of Human Stress, 6,* 15-22.

Gorsuch, R.L. & Key, M.K. (1974). Abnormalities of pregnancy as a function of anxiety and life stress. *Psychosomatic Medicine, 36,* 4, 352-362.

Helper, M.M., Cohen, R.L., Beiteman, E.T., & Eaton, L.F. (1968). Life-events and acceptance of pregnancy. *Journal of Psychosomatic Research, 12,* 183-188.

Jones, A.C. (1978). Life changes and psychological distress as predictors of pregnancy outcome. *Psychosomatic Medicine, 40,* 5, 402-412.

Jones, A.C. (1975). Psychological assessment as an adjunct to obstetrical screening of high risk pregnancies: an exploratory study. *Dis. Abs. Intl., 36,* 1, 445-B.

Kuhn, T.S. (1962). *The structure of scientific revolutions.* Chicago: University of Chicago Press.

Nuckolls, K.B. (1971). Psychosocial assets, life crisis and the prognosis of pregnancy. *Dis. Abs. Intl., 31,* 5-B, 2796-B.

Pedhazur, E.H. (1982). *Multiple regression in behavioral research* (2nd ed., p. 582). New York: Holt, Rinehart and Winston.

Rahe, R.H., Meyer, M., Smith, M., Kjaer, G., & Holmes, T.H. (1964). Social stress and illness onset. *Journal Psychosomatic Research, 8,* 35-44.

Schaie, K.W. (1965). A general model for the study of developmental problems. *Psychological Bulletin, 64,* 2, 92-107.

Schwartz, J.L. (1973). A study of the relationship between maternal life change events and premature delivery. Unpublished Master's Thesis. University of Washington.

Thurlow, H.J. (1967). General susceptibility to illness: A selective review. *Canadian Medical Association Journal, 97,* 1397-1404.

3

Application Of Stress Scales To A Childbearing Year Program

Introduction

Prenatal care is considered an essential element in health care of childbearing women. The types of prenatal care, however, are legion. Most emphasize routine office visits to a health-care provider, and some, in the event of problems, prescribe a battery of laboratory and other technological procedures designed to monitor the course of pregnancy. Some few others emphasize nutrition, physical exercise, and/or preparation for labor and delivery.

Over the past 10 years, the concept of risk identification and categorization of women according to their degree of risk based on medical and obstetrical conditions, has become a recognized part of prenatal care. The predictive accuracy of the various risk indexes has been somewhat disappointing. At the same time there has been increased awareness of the idea of risk reduction and health maintenance, and promotion during the childbearing period. Although both concepts have been documented in practice and in research literature, less attention has been paid to development of high-level wellness than to high-risk care.

The Childbearing Year approach to preparation for childbirth and early parenting constituted a major advance in the field. Traditional approaches to preparation for childbirth have mainly involved classes during the last part of pregnancy, with didactic presentations of factual information in the rather narrow range of preparation for labor, and some skill development in breathing and relaxation techniques.

The phrase, "The Childbearing Year," was coined in the early 1970's by Peg Beals, past president of the International Childbirth Education Association. It refers to the time period from conception to three months after the delivery. The concept was developed out of an awareness of the need to assist expectant couples and new parents throughout the whole year of childbearing, not just at the end of pregnancy through the early postpartum period.

The concept of a Childbearing Year Program at the College of Nursing, University of Utah, was first implemented in November, 1977. Developed and conducted by faculty and graduate nurse-midwifery students, it was, and is, reflective of nurse-midwives' commitment to provision of holistic care of their clients. There were a number of reasons why we thought that such a program had great potential for facilitating high-level wellness within childbearing families.

1. The number of direct contact hours with couples in the Childbearing Year Program far exceeds that of usual health system contacts during childbearing. The average physician probably spends a maximum total of about six hours with an essentially normal woman during her pregnancy, labor and delivery, and the postpartum period. Contact with the woman's partner may be confined to a few office visits and a brief encounter at delivery. Our CBY program involves a series of 13 two-hour group sessions, 4 occuring in early pregnancy, 5 in late pregnancy, and 4 within the first six weeks after birth. This is a total of 26 contact hours. A maximum of 12 couples (usually 6-8) is enrolled in each series. The CBY program therefore, provides a considerable supplement of time in addition to usual health care provider contacts.

2. The couple in this phase of their life experience is particularly open to learning and behavior change relative to a quality pregnancy experience, and health maintenance and promotion. The CBY program, therefore, provides a unique opportunity to facilitate positive personal health practices during and beyond the childbearing year. Ultimately, it is these personal health practices that have the greatest potential for improving and maintaining individual and family health in our society.

3. The major thrust of the CBY Program is on developing high-level wellness in the family unit through information, skill development, and increased confidence and motivation to be an active participant in one's own health care. Although the classical professional response to the needs of childbearing couples has been the proliferation of specialized knowledge and powerful techniques for specific problems, much of this information has been relatively unavailable to expectant couples and new parents. The nurse childbith educator however, through a comprehensive CBY program, can provide information from various disciplines applicable to the many different needs of this time period. Such a program enables the

group leader to be a strong and consistent support person who has access to the specialized knowledge of nursing, obstetrics, gynecology, pediatrics, and the social sciences, and who may be a referring source to other professionals.

Our program goal was to enhance high-level wellness in the pregnant woman and the new family. Therefore, we wanted to develop an assessment and teaching matrix that would address as many potentially relevent elements as we could identify.

We believed that the PIPAS scales and research findings would materially assist us in individualizing our approach to the expectant couples. Our two-pronged effort involves individual assessment followed by group discussion during the class sessions.

Assessment Of The Childbearing Couple

Each expectant couple is given an assessment packet at the first class session in the Early Pregnancy series (Appendix A). They are requested to complete it individually, and mail it back before the next class session, in a preaddressed stamped envelope. This packet contains health assessment questionnaires, the stress profile questionnaires, and physical fitness forms. The nutrition assessment forms are returned at the second class since they take the full seven days to complete. A secretary prepares the profiles based on the mailed-in materials, and they are reviewed and completed by the group leader prior to the second class. An abbreviated second packet, with portions of the PIPAS profile, is completed later in pregnancy so that PIPAS data is available for all three trimesters of pregnancy.

A unique focus of the program is that assessment information and teaching are geared to the partner and his health and well-being as well as to that of his wife. His needs are seen as distinct, in addition to his role vis-a-vis the woman. Although we welcome and include women without partners, the majority of our clients bring a support person to the classes, such as a female family member or a friend. All information is treated confidentially. The individuals do sign a release enabling us to use the data, without identification, for research purposes as well as for their immediate benefit within the confines of the classes.

The Childbearing Year Program

Group leaders are registered nurses. Some of them are nurses from the community who have taken our continuing education program to prepare childbirth educators to teach a Childbearing Year approach, and some are graduate students in nurse-midwifery who are required to take several courses in preparation for childbirth education as a part of their master's degree program. The concepts, though, can be utilized by anyone prepared to provide health services to childbearing families.

Several grants from the March of Dimes and the Division of Nursing, Bureau of Health Professions, have enabled the curriculum development and research activities reported here. During the grant periods we have (a) developed a data bank for information obtained from couples as they progress through the program, (b) analyzed portions of the data, (c) developed curriculum and materials for each of the 13 classes in the series, and (d) produced a slide/tape as a motivational trigger for the nutrition portion of the program. This media also has an accompanying instructors guide for utilization of the Agnes Higgins Intervention Method for Nutritional Rehabilitation During Pregnancy (Foster, 1981).

In addition to the childbirth related topics considered in the Early Pregnancy, Late Pregnancy, and Early Parenting series, specific focus has been placed on stress reduction, nutrition, physical fitness, personal habits hazards reduction, and active participation in health care decisions with the woman's health care provider. We believe that all of the above topics have potential for reducing the physical as well as the emotional stresses of childbearing.

This high-level wellness focus of the program begins in the four classes of the Early Pregnancy Series and is seen as the most critical and important segment of our Childbearing Year program. We believe that these classes, together with sound prenatal obstetrical care by qualified health care providers, have potential for preventing many problems and stresses that may occur later in pregnancy, at delivery, or in the newborn and postpartum periods. Also, the enthusiasm and inerest of the expectant couples have encouraged us in our belief that what we are offering is meaningful and useful to them.

The first class consists of information concerning maternal and fetal changes and developments, and is designed to promote the concepts that

(a) the fetus is a real human being requiring maternal assistance for optimal growth and development, and (b) the quality of the pregnancy experience and health of the expectant mother can be positively influenced by her actions. Comfort measures for common problems are taught.

The second class focuses on the actions the mother can take to build a healthy baby. Topics include maternal-placental relationships; avoidance of personal and environmental hazards believed to affect health such as drugs, chemicals, infections, hyperthermia; and ensuring physical fitness. A considerable portion of this class is spent on discussion of stress reduction. A more detailed presentation of this aspect is discussed below.

The third class is designed to develop informed consumerism. Rights, responsibilities, and options are discussed. Getting the most out of prenatal visits, costs and purchases, and danger signs to physical and emotional health during pregnancy are also addressed.

The fourth class of the series is about nutrition. This class is based on the premise that an accurate assessment of individual status and need is prerequisite to any discussion of appropriate types and amounts of foods in pregnancy. Therefore, the seven-day diet analysis, based on the food-intake records, forms the basis of the data for this class.

Information and class discussions are directed toward specific risk reduction activities and motivation to engage in practices that will enhance the well-being of the individuals and their developing baby. The health maintenance and promotion concepts of the Early Pregnancy Series are reinforced throughout the Late Pregnancy and Early Parenting Series, with appropriate additional content and application. The remainder of this chapter will present the program and data as it relates to stress and pregnancy.

Stress And Pregnancy: The CBY Program

Individual profile feedback is given to the individual at the second class session. Pooled data from previous classes provide a normative group against which the individual may compare his/her profile. The group leader utilizes her knowledge of the class members profiles to direct the discussion in relation to individual and group needs, without breaching confidentiality. We view the group leader as a resource for the couple to help them cope more comfortably and capably with their experience by helping them to identify problem areas, recognize their significance, and plan strategies for meeting their individual needs.

Group members are encouraged to share strategies for stress reduction that they have found useful. Unproductive or dangerous responses to stress (such as anti-social behavior, excessive alcohol intake, etc.) are identified and discussed.

The following specific strategies are encouraged:

1. Recognize the stress by bringing it to cognitive awareness. For example, a profile of the PIPAS scales has helped individuals to pinpoint specific stresses. Although an individual may feel his employment causes emotional stress, seeing it verified through a high score on the profile sheet, based on his/her response to a series of work related questions, often brings a sense of relief in its specific identification as a stressor. Cognitive awareness is a prerequisite to initiating the process of conscious behavioral response for stress reduction. In addition, recognition of symptoms of a stress response will bring it to cognitive awareness. The more cognitive and conceptual control one has over one's life events (i.e., understanding their potential impact), the greater the potential for changing behavior, reducing the subsequent symptoms and improving pregnancy outcome.

2. Talk about the stress with a supportive person. Many couples describe a great sense of relief whenever they can both label and describe their stresses to a caring listener. We encourage the couple to be supportive to each other in their needs to express their problems verbally and receive nurturing responses.

3. Utilize both general relaxation techniques and on-the-spot relaxation whenever a stress response is identified. We encourage the couple to practice the progressive relaxation techniques learned in class at least once a day for a minimum of 10 minutes. In addition, we teach them to carry out exhalation relaxation (a deep sighing breath with deliberate muscle tension release during exhalation) whenever they are aware of experiencing a stress response. In addition to the general progressive relaxation technique and the Lamaze-based dissociation relaxation taught for use in labor, we also teach Sheila Kitzinger's touch relaxation approach to increase couple communication, and reduce general and

specific stresses (Kitzinger, 1977).

4. Use rhythmic motion. The prophylactic and therapeutic use of a rocking chair for at least a 10-minute time period daily is encouraged. Couples are encouraged to obtain a rocking chair early in pregnancy and use it before as well as after the baby is born.

5. Use aerobic exercise as a means of endorphin release for an increased sense of well-being, as well as a means of physical fitness development or maintenance. A brisk walk for 30 minutes four-to-six times a week, or as needed for a specific stress response, or swimming laps for the same time period are safe, appropriate aerobic activities generally available to most pregnant women. The value of aerobic exercise for life, for both the man and the woman, is also emphasized.

6. Simplify your life, if you are stress vulnerable. Stress-vulnerable individuals attract stresses, have a poor regulation of stress mechanisms, are not skilled at predicting and controlling the consequences of stresses, and tend to lead a crisis lifestyle. This is a particular problem for persons striving in the professions. Both physical and emotional energy is required due to the state of pregnancy. Every additional stress detracts from the quality of the pregnancy experience. The stress potential of even pleasant new experiences can place inordinate demands upon the system. Couples need to orient themselves to decreasing other life stresses during this time. This may be done by not taking on any new, additional tasks or other life-style changes (stresses) if at all possible.

The Stress Data: The CBY Program

Demographic Data:

There are 178 women whose longitudinal data are reported in this series. The major source of information about the program was through friends, health-care provider, or a television announcement. All but 12% were in their first or second trimester of pregnancy when they registered. The women ranged in age from 15 to 36 years with a mean age of 24 and a standard deviation of 4.7 years. Ninety-two percent were married. Seventy percent of the women had at least one year of college education. Seventeen percent had a family income less than $7,000 a year, and 22% had an income of over $21,000 a year. Twenty-six percent were obtaining care from a certified nurse-midwife, and the remainder were being seen by a physician. Seventy-nine percent of the women were primigravidas. Of the 59 multigravidas, 24 reported a previous delivery of from one to four infants weighing under 2500 grams (5½ lbs.). This may have been a motivating factor for at least half of the multigravidas who enrolled in the program.

Sixty percent reported that this was a planned pregnancy. When asked the ease of this pregnancy so far, 34% stated that it was easier than they had expected, 35% stated it was as they had expected, and 38% said that it was harder than they had expected.

PIPAS Profile:

There were 138 women who completed the PIPAS profile relative to their first trimester of pregnancy. The remainder of the women registered after the early pregnancy series. There were 127 who completed second-trimester data while third-trimester data is available for only 79 of these women. Most of the drop-off was due to failure to return the later packet, and in some instances early delivery or moving away precluded completion of the last-trimester data.

Symptom Proneness:

As indicated in Chapter 1, the Symptom Proneness Index consists of 32 physical symptoms. The women were asked to indicate those symptoms that they had experienced within the past 10 years. A comparison of this score with the health history information aided us in identifying those very few individuals who had a number of disease/illness entities responsible for a high score, but probably not related to a stress response per se.

The normative PIPAS data based on 255 second-trimester women showed a mean score of 6.47 items with a standard deviation of 3.91 items. Our childbearing year sample of 138 women had a mean score of 7.3 items with a standard deviation of 4.6 items. The range of 0 to 25 items indicates great variability among the class participants. This is probably a reflection of the heterogeneity of our groups (Table 1).

Pregnancy Symptoms:

One measure of the quality of a pregnancy is the number of difficult symptoms that are associated with the pregnancy. The set of severe and frequent pregnancy symptoms developed in the PIPAS Project were given to the CBY participants. It may be seen in Table 1 that the mean number of items scored out of 54 total items from the six scales was approximately the same during the first two trimesters (13.2 and 13.6 respectively), and increased slightly to 15.6 during the third trimester.

The information on the individual scales from both the PIPAS project and the CBY data gives us the first documented perspective of the physical pregnancy experience. This information may be of particular use to the clinician in evaluating whether a symptom in a particular client represents a usual frequency at that point in gestation, or may be indicative of a possible problem. In addition to suggestions to the woman regarding how to manage/reduce the symptom for maximum confort, it may also be reassuring for her to know that a certain percentage of women experience that symptom at that point in the pregnancy.

The personal profile sheet (Figure 1), used in the CBY program, indicate to both the group leader and the woman whether her total number of identified symptoms in a particular system-grouping falls within the normative range of one standard deviation, or whether she is in the top 15% of women, i.e., above one standard deviation, and therefore presumably at greater risk. This risk could be an indication of current medical/obstetrical high-risk conditions and/or indicative of stress that could have an impact on her health status, quality of pregnancy, and/or outcome. In combination with other aspects of the PIPAS profile, a woman could be categorized generally as to her level of stress and risk.

Gastrointestinal Symptoms:

The nine items in this scale show variations in pattern throughout pregnancy (Table 2). The data show a slight decline in gastrointestinal symptoms overall, throughout the three trimesters. The PIPAS mean of 3.248 with a standard deviation of 2.199, is slightly higher than the CBY group in the second trimester, but about the same as that group in the first trimester.

TABLE 1
Summary Of PIPAS Data

		First Trimester N = 138			Second Trimester N = 127			Third Trimester N = 79		
Scale	N Items	Mean	S.D.	Range	Mean	S.D.	Range	Mean	S.D.	Range
Symptom Proneness	32	7.3	4.6	0-25	-	-	-	-	-	-
Pregnancy Symptoms										
Gastrointestinal Symptoms	9	3.1	1.9	0-9	2.1	1.9	0-9	2.0	1.6	0-9
General Adaptational Stress Symptoms	9	3.9	2.3	0-9	3.1	2.4	0-9	3.3	2.5	0-9
Reproductive Symptoms	9	3.5	1.5	0-8	3.4	1.9	0-8	3.5	1.6	0-8
Neuromuscular Symptoms	9	.85	1.3	0-8	1.5	1.7	0-8	2.7	2.3	0-9
Skin Symptoms	9	.83	1.2	0-9	1.2	1.3	0-8	1.5	1.5	0-9
Cardiovascular-Respiratory Symptoms	9	1.0	1.4	0-7	1.9	1.8	0-8	2.8	1.9	0-7
TOTAL Symptoms Without Cornell Psychiatric Index	54	13.2	6.8	0-48	13.6	8.4	0-50	15.6	8.8	0-40
Cornell Psychiatric Index	20	2.2	3.1	0-19	2.5	3.7	0-19	2.3	4.1	0-19

Life Change Units	N Items	6-12 Months Ago N = 139 Mean	S.D.	Range	0-6 Months Ago N = 139 Mean	S.D.	Range	Since Last Report N = 31 Mean	S.D.	Range
Social Stress	9	.77	1.2	0-8	1.1	2.2	0-7	.58	.84	0-3
Work Stress	9	1.2	1.5	0-7	2.5	2.7	0-9	.84	1.4	0-5
Family Stress	9	.94	1.3	0-6	1.7	1.8	0-7	1.0	1.3	0-4
Financial Stress	9	1.5	1.6	0-6	2.7	2.0	0-8	1.9	1.9	0-6
Lifestyle Stress	9	1.5	1.7	0-8	3.1	2.1	0-8	2.3	1.8	0-6
Personal Habits Stress	9	1.4	1.9	0-9	4.4	2.7	0-9	3.6	2.7	0-9

FIGURE 1. PIPAS Profile Pregnancy, Illness Proneness and Stress

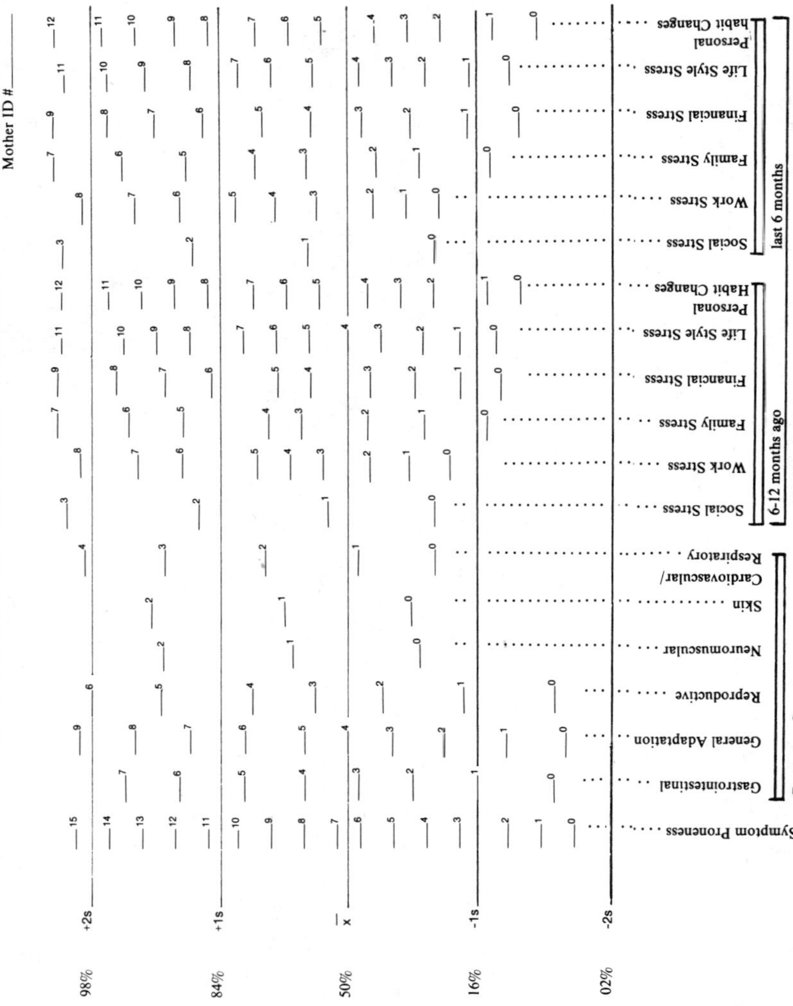

TABLE 2

Gastrointestinal Symptoms
CBY Females — Evening Series

	1st Trimester N = 130					2nd Trimester N = 127					3rd Trimester N = 79				
	No		Yes		Missing Data	No		Yes		Missing Data	No		Yes		Missing Data
	N	%	N	%	N	N	%	N	%	N	N	%	N	%	N
Loss of Appetite	85	62	53	38	40	111	87	16	13	51	69	87	10	13	99
Frequent Dry Mouth/Bad Breath	102	74	36	26	40	91	72	36	28	51	59	75	20	25	99
Frequent Constipation	108	78	30	22	40	96	76	31	24	51	57	72	22	28	99
Certain Foods Bother	64	46	74	54	40	91	72	36	28	51	52	66	27	44	99
Nausea/Morning Sickness	34	25	104	75	40	101	80	26	20	51	68	54	11	46	99
Vomiting	122	88	16	12	40	114	90	13	10	51	76	96	3	4	99
Heartburn	115	83	23	17	40	88	69	39	31	51	38	48	41	52	99
Stomach Cramps	110	80	28	20	40	105	83	22	17	51	66	84	13	16	99
Crave Certain Foods	86	82	52	38	40	84	66	43	44	51	60	76	19	24	99

Gastrointestinal Total Score:

	1st Trimester	2nd Trimester	3rd Trimester
Mean	3.1	2.1	2.0
SD	1.9	1.9	1.6
Range	0-9	0-9	0-9

The most frequently occurring symptom, Nausea/Morning Sickness, occurred in 75% of women during the first trimester, but dropped to 20% and 14% respectively, in the second and third trimesters. Therefore, its occurrence later in pregnancy should probably be evaluated more carefully by the clinician in relation to other variables of health status. The item, Certain Foods Bother, was next in frequency of occurrence with 54% of women reporting this symptom in the first trimester. There was a drop to 28% of women in the second trimester reporting this symptom, and a slight rise to 34% in the third trimester. Loss of Appetite was noticed by 38% of women in the first trimester, with a sharp drop in the occurrence of this symptom to 13% in the second and third trimesters.

The beginning of the second trimester seems to be an appropriate time to encourage the increase in the amount of protein and calories necessary for an optimal pregnancy weight gain. It is interesting to note that Crave Certain Foods increased from 38% to 44% during the first two trimesters, and then dropped to 24%.

Approximately one-third of the women were troubled by Frequent Constipation throughout their pregnancy. The symptom Heartburn showed a steady increase from 17% through 31% to 52% in the last trimester. The least-frequently occurring items, Frequent Dry Mouth/Bad Breath/Vomiting, and Stomach Cramps occurred in less than a quarter of the women, and did not vary markedly throughout pregnancy.

General Adaptational Stress Symptoms:

There is a slight decline in the total for this scale during the second trimester, with a slight rise in the third, but not back, to the level of the first trimester (Table 3). This indicates that the major adjustments to the pregnancy do take place during the first trimester, with the middle trimester more quiescent and the third demanding some additional adjustments. As in the GI Scale, the second trimester mean for the PIPAS data (3.936, SD 2.510) more closely reflects the first trimester data of the CBY group.

The three energy/fatigue items: Felt Persistently Tired, Not Much Energy, and Tired in A.M. were reported by 63% to 70% of the women during the first trimester, dropped to 37% to 50% during the second trimester and rose slightly in the third trimester. The first trimester

TABLE 3

General Adaptational Distress
CBY Females — Evening Series

	1st Trimester N = 138					2nd Trimester N = 127					3rd Trimester N = 79				
	No		Yes		Missing Data	No		Yes		Missing Data	No		Yes		Missing Data
	N	%	N	%	N	N	%	N	%	N	N	%	N	%	N
Frequent Frightening Dreams	114	83	24	17	40	103	81	24	19	51	65	82	14	17	99
Felt Persistently Tired	42	30	96	70	40	75	59	52	41	51	47	59	32	41	99
Not Much Energy	47	34	91	66	40	64	50	63	50	51	34	43	45	57	99
Increased Nervous Irritability	83	60	55	40	40	85	67	42	33	51	51	65	28	35	99
Sensitive to Light/Sounds/Smells	78	57	60	43	40	83	65	44	35	51	55	70	24	30	99
Trouble Getting to Sleep	110	80	28	20	40	90	71	37	29	51	44	64	35	36	99
Trouble Staying Asleep	111	80	27	20	40	85	67	42	33	51	34	43	45	57	99
Tired in A.M.	51	37	87	63	40	80	63	47	37	51	41	52	38	48	99
Headaches	93	67	45	33	40	94	74	32	26	51	69	87	10	13	99
General Adaptational Distress Total Score:															
Mean			3.9			3.1					3.3				
SD			2.3			2.4					2.5				
Range			0-9			0-9					0-9				

symptoms are probably a reflection of physiologic adjustments while the third-trimester increase is probably due to the increasing physical load of the pregnancy. The number of women reporting the symptom Headaches showed a steady drop during the three trimesters from 33% to 13%.

Sensitive to Light/Sounds/Smells and Increased Nervous Irritability also decreased slightly as the pregnancy progressed. Trouble Getting to Sleep and Trouble Staying Asleep increased throughout the pregnancy for one-third to one-half of the women. Approximately 17% to 19% of the women reported Frequent Frightening Dreams throughout their pregnancy. The range of from zero to nine items reported indicates the variability between women, and the sensitivity of the scale in identifying women who are having problems adjusting to the pregnancy.

Reproductive Symptoms.

The reproductive system symptoms remained fairly constant. The PIPAS mean of 2.593, SD 1.695, was slightly less than the 3.4 and 3.5 means reported by the CBY women (Table 4). This particular symptom set does not show strong covariations with other variables, with the result that a different set of reproductive system symptoms should probably be developed in the future.

Painful Breasts and Tingling in the Breasts have a sharp drop in occurrence after the first trimester, and fewer women report Increased Breast Size as the pregnancy progresses. Uterine Contractions and Sharp Abdominal Pain show progressive increase in incidence throughout the pregnancy. There is a marked increase in reporting of Feel Stretched out of Shape as the pregnancy progresses, and a lesser but progressive increase in Increased Vaginal Discharge.

Frequent Urination, reported by 72% of women in the first trimester, decreases slightly in the second trimester to 63% and rises again to 80% of the women during the third trimester. Burning During Urination, a pathologic symptom indicative of urinary tract infection, is present in 6% to 10% of women throughout pregnancy. All of these items are well correlated with both physiologic as well as physical changes throughout pregnancy, and therefore are probably not very useful indicators of variance in stress responses in pregnancy.

TABLE 4

Reproductive System Symptoms
CBY Females — Evening Series

	1st Trimester N = 138					2nd Trimester N = 127					3rd Trimester N = 79				
	No		Yes		Missing Data	No		Yes		Missing Data	No		Yes		Missing Data
	N	%	N	%	N	N	%	N	%	N	N	%	N	%	N
Increased Vaginal Discharge	96	70	42	30	40	86	68	41	32	51	49	62	30	38	99
Painful Breasts	53	38	85	62	40	92	72	35	28	51	74	94	5	6	99
Tingling in Breasts	92	67	46	33	40	110	87	17	13	51	69	87	10	13	99
Increased Breast Size	33	24	105	76	40	40	31	87	69	51	41	52	38	48	99
Uterine Contractions	118	86	20	14	40	91	72	36	28	51	47	59	32	41	99
Sharp Abdominal Pain	95	69	43	31	40	67	53	60	47	51	35	44	44	56	99
Feel Stretched Out of Shape	114	83	24	17	40	72	57	55	43	51	19	24	60	76	99
Frequent Urination	39	28	99	72	40	47	37	80	63	51	16	20	63	80	99
Burning During Urination	130	94	8	6	40	120	94	7	6	51	71	90	7	10	99

Reproductive System Total Score:

	1st Trimester	2nd Trimester	3rd Trimester
Mean	3.5	3.4	3.5
SD	1.5	1.9	1.6
Range	0-8	0-8	0-8

Neuromuscular Symptoms:

CBY women reported a greater mean total of neuromuscular symptoms than did the PIPAS normative group. The PIPAS mean was .646, SD 1.026, compared with an increasing number reported throughout pregnancy in the CBY group, i.e., .85, 1.5 and 2.7, respectively. However, it may be seen that this group of symptoms occurs much less frequently (Table 5).

Low Backache was the most commonly reported symptom in this scale, increasing from 28% in the first trimester, through 40% in the second, to 53% in the third trimester. All of the other symptoms were reported at less than a 14% incidence in the first trimester to about 33% of the group reporting these symptoms generally, in the third trimester. The single exception was Pain in the Rib Cage, which increased from a low of 4% and 17%, respectively, in the first two trimesters, to a high of 44% in the third trimester.

Skin Symptoms:

Skin symptoms followed the same general pattern as the neuromuscular symptoms, with a PIPAS mean slightly lower than the CBY data, i.e., .640 with a standard deviation of .918. There was a small increase throughout pregnancy from .83 in the first trimester to a high of 1.5 in the third trimester (Table 6). Although the number of items reported is quite small, it is significant to note that the range was from 0 to 9 symptoms, indicating variability and sensitivity of the scale.

The most frequently reported symptom was Stretch Marks, which were noted by 14% in the first trimester, 27% in the second trimester, and 44% of the women by the third trimester of pregnancy. The next most common symptom was Itching Skin, with a 17% incidence in the first trimester, 28% incidence in the second trimester, and a 38% reported incidence in the third trimester.

All of the other seven skin symptoms occurred infrequently, from 3% to 11% in the first trimester to a high of 8% to 24% in the third trimester. Five of the seven had a sequential increase in incidence. Definite Rashes and Bruise Easily increased in the second trimester and dropped in the third trimester.

TABLE 5

Neuromuscular Symptoms
CBY Females — Evening Series

	1st Trimester N = 138					2nd Trimester N = 127					3rd Trimester N = 79				
	No		Yes		Missing Data	No		Yes		Missing Data	No		Yes		Missing Data
	N	%	N	%	N	N	%	N	%	N	N	%	N	%	N
Muscle Cramps	131	95	7	5	40	101	80	26	20	51	53	67	25	33	99
Low Backache	99	72	39	28	40	76	60	51	40	51	37	47	40	53	99
Stiff or Sore Joints	128	93	10	7	40	114	90	13	10	51	56	71	21	29	99
Aching Arms/Legs	119	86	19	14	40	105	83	22	17	51	53	67	24	33	99
Numbness in Arms/Legs	132	96	6	4	40	115	91	12	9	51	65	82	12	18	99
Weakness in Arms/Legs	130	94	8	6	40	115	91	12	9	51	61	77	16	23	99
Tendency to Drop Things	121	88	17	12	40	103	81	24	19	51	56	71	21	29	99
Pains in Rib Cage	132	96	6	4	40	114	83	13	17	51	44	56	33	44	99
Difficulty Walking	133	96	5	4	40	109	86	18	14	51	51	65	26	35	99

Reproductive System Total Score:

	1st Trimester	2nd Trimester	3rd Trimester
Mean	0.85	1.5	2.7
SD	1.3	1.7	2.3
Range	0-8	0-8	0-9

Cardiovascular/Respiratory Symptoms:

The last of the pregnancy scales, Cardiovascular/Respiratory Symptoms, also followed the pattern of Skin and Neuromuscular. The PIPAS mean was 1.090 with a standard deviation of 1.428. The CBY data increased throughout the pregnancy with mean scores of 1.0, 1.9 and 2.8, respectively (Table 7). The range of symptoms reported was from zero to seven.

Eight of the nine symptoms showed an increased incidence as the three trimesters progressed. Frequent Cough only occurred in 5% in the first trimester and leveled off at 9% in the last two trimesters. The occurrence of Stuffy Nose increased from 26% to 41%. Frequent Shortness of Breath and Sleep on 2 or More Pillows both increased, from 7% and 6%, to 49% and 43%, respectively.

Swelling in Ankles/Leg and Swelling in Hands/Face increased from 6% and 1%, to 39% and 27% respectively. Feel Heart Pounding increased from 18% to 37% by the last trimester. Frequent Colds showed a small increase from 11% to 15% at the end of pregnancy. Frequently Hot/Flushed increased from 11% in the first trimester to 21% in the second, and 35% in the third trimester.

Concordance Between Couples Regarding Pregnancy Symptoms:

As noted earlier, the woman's partner also is encouraged to fill out the assessment packet. While the Symptom Proneness, CPI and Lifestyle Changes relate to him directly, the Pregnancy Symptoms Scales are a reflection of his perception of whether his wife is experiencing the given symptom.

His score of his perceptions are plotted against his wife's report, on the same profile sheet. This enables the group leader and the couple to note the number of items in each scale scored by both husband and wife, the items scored by the wife only (not known to the husband), and the items scored by the husband only (not reported by the wife).

In characterizing husbands and their relations to their pregnant wives, we are noting that there is a continuum from "sensitizers" to "repressors," with the majority of men somewhere in the middle. The husband who is a "sensitizer" is the type who over-estimates the symptoms his pregnant wife has; the "repressor" tends to ignore or explain away as non-

TABLE 6

Skin Symptoms
CBY Females — Evening Series

	1st Trimester N = 138					2nd Trimester N = 127					3rd Trimester N = 79				
	No		Yes		Missing Data	No		Yes		Missing Data	No		Yes		Missing Data
	N	%	N	%	N	N	%	N	%	N	N	%	N	%	N
Hands Often Sweaty	134	97	4	3	40	120	94	7	6	51	70	89	9	11	99
Definite Rashes	125	91	13	9	40	110	87	17	13	51	72	91	6	9	99
Itching Skin	115	83	23	17	40	92	72	35	28	51	49	62	29	38	99
Perspire a Great Deal	123	89	15	11	40	110	87	17	13	51	60	76	18	24	99
Skin Blotches	131	95	7	5	40	112	88	15	12	51	67	85	11	15	99
Marked Hair Changes	123	89	15	11	40	112	88	15	12	51	68	86	10	14	99
Skin Infections	133	96	5	4	40	123	97	4	3	51	73	92	5	8	99
Bruise Easily	126	91	12	9	40	113	89	14	11	51	73	92	5	8	99
Stretch Marks	118	86	20	14	40	93	73	34	27	51	44	56	34	44	99

Skin Total Score		1st Trimester	2nd Trimester	3rd Trimester
	Mean	0.83	1.2	1.5
	SD	1.2	1.3	1.5
	Range	0-9	0-9	0-9

TABLE 7

Cardiovascular — Respiratory Symptoms
CBY Females — Evening Series

	1st Trimester N = 138					2nd Trimester N = 127					3rd Trimester N = 79				
	No		Yes		Missing Data	No		Yes		Missing Data	No		Yes		Missing Data
	N	%	N	%	N	N	%	N	%	N	N	%	N	%	N
Feel Heart Pounding	113	82	25	18	40	90	71	37	29	51	50	63	27	37	99
Frequent Shortness of Breath	128	93	10	7	40	89	70	38	30	51	40	51	37	49	99
Sleep on 2 or More Pillows	130	94	8	6	40	101	80	26	20	51	45	57	32	43	99
Frequent Colds	123	89	15	11	40	109	86	18	14	51	67	85	10	15	99
Stuffy Nose	102	74	36	26	40	80	63	47	37	51	47	59	30	41	99
Frequent Cough	131	95	7	5	40	115	91	12	9	51	72	91	5	9	99
Swelling in Ankles/Legs	130	94	8	6	40	107	84	20	16	51	48	61	29	39	99
Swelling in Hands/Face	136	99	2	1	40	120	94	7	6	51	58	73	19	27	99
Frequently Hot/Flushed	123	89	15	11	40	100	79	27	21	51	51	65	30	35	99

Cardiovascular — Respiratory Total Score

	1st Trimester	2nd Trimester	3rd Trimester
Mean	1.0	1.9	2.8
SD	1.4	1.8	1.9
Range	0-7	0-8	0-7

significant most of the symptoms of his pregnant wife.

While in the initial phases of pregnancy, the "sensitizer" husband will closely monitor his wife's reaction to the pregnancy and thus have quick, strong empathic bonds. Over the long haul, however, he tends to be an obsessive worrier. He tends to be hypochondriacal where the pregnancy is concerned, and because he is not realistically oriented, he may be less capable of sustained support of his wife.

In contrast to the "sensitizer," the "repressor" may not entertain in consciousness, without much anxiety, the difficulties his wife is undergoing, and thus tends to isolate himself from knowledge of her symptoms. Possibly, facing symptoms he neither understands nor can do anything about makes him feel powerless and helpless. Thus, the tendency is to define the childbearing processes as exclusively "women's business."

The strong reaction we get in some classes is that the husband really has little knowledge of the symptoms of his wife and becomes annoyed when he is expected to know what she is going through. In some cases he may refuse to answer that part of the survey which asks what symptoms his wife has during a particular phase of pregnancy. We believe, however, that using this technique may be an opening wedge of understanding for many men regarding the psychological and physiological changes which occur in pregnancy.

The information couples obtain from these data facilitates group discussion about the ways couples may become more empathic and mutually supportive. For the husband, attendance at prenatal classes, participation in the labor, witnessing the delivery, instruction in the care of the infant, and help in the immediate postpartum care of the baby, all contribute to the attachment process between the various family members. Sensitive concern for, and consideration of his physical symptoms, views, and concerns relative to the pregnancy facilitate his own growth and development through this important life experience.

In some instances, the lack of concordance in reporting symptoms is simply due to lack of communication between the couple. Such communication is encouraged within the class framework in a number of ways: through discussion, role modeling of some of the class members, mutual feedback during the exercise sessions, and through use of touch relaxation by both partners with each other.

Cornell Psychiatric Index:

In the initial CBY study the 20 items of the Cornell Psychiatric Index were compared with the normative PIPAS data. Based on 255 second trimester women the mean score was 2.3882 with a standard deviation of 2.8853. The CBY data was comparable with means in each of the three trimesters of 2.2, 2.5 and 2.3 respectively (Table 1). We did have a range of from 0 to 19 items scored by individuals.

Although we believe that the psychiatric variables don't cause but are probably intensifiers affecting coping, we were not sure just how to handle this information in feedback to individuals. It appeared that scores of 3, 4, or 5 items were probably representative of the woman's emotional changes in pregnancy that made such material more available to her consciousness. Higher scores probably represented a need for counseling. However, because of the sensitive nature of the data and the uncertainty we had about how to give appropriate feedback, we decided not to use the CPI in preparing the individual profiles. To date, this data has been used only in the research analysis.

Life Change Units:

As in the Pregnancy Symptoms Scales, our concern for individuals was focused on those profiles where one or more of the scales had a score greater than one standard deviation above the mean, or in the top 15% of individuals reporting the items of a given scale. Obviously, those scales with higher reliability coefficients would be more useful in predicting association with other variables. For prediction of pregnancy symptoms the most important scores were (a) personal habits changes and (b) family changes.

The couples found the LCU section of the PIPAS profile very interesting and helpful. They could verify that indeed a high score was reflective of what they were experiencing in relation to stress in that scale domain. Their profile became a tool for decision making in relation to stress reduction, when it was seen that a complex of high scores in several scale areas might mean increased risk relative to health and the quality of the pregnancy experience.

Table 1 gives the data for the six scale domains in three time periods. The 6-12 Months Ago and the 0-6 Months Ago data was filled out as part of the Early Pregnancy Series. The Since Last Report Data was requested from some couples during their Late Pregnancy Series.

It is interesting to note that the highest mean scores were found in the time period 0-6 Months Ago, reflecting their experience in the first two trimesters of pregnancy. For a number of couples this time period was one in which both the adjustments of marriage and pregnancy were taking place. The 6-12 Month Ago period for the newly married reflected their more orderly existence as single people and the 0 to 6 month period represented the tremendous adjustments they were experiencing currently. We would like to think that the lower scores for the 31 individuals late in pregnancy are reflective of their efforts to regularize their lives after obtaining the information from the CBY classes.

All the pregnancy symptoms that a person reports for the first two trimesters have been combined into an index, called QPREG, quality of pregnancy. A path diagram of a number of variables as they contribute to this quality of pregnancy index was constructed (Figure 2). This path diagram will be discussed below.

Psychological Symptoms:

Not only do the number of annoying pregnancy symptoms a person has affect the quality of her pregnancy, but also the psychological tasks of the pregnancy. The pregnancy process is thought to have five tasks for resolving: (a) reactions to being pregnant, (b) reactions to the hormonal adjustments of the pregnancy, and to nausea and vomiting, (c) reactions to the quickening and the psychological reaction to motherhood, (d) reactions to the physiological strain of the late pregnancy, and (e) the calm, lassitude that overcomes women in the last few weeks of pregnancy.

The first two events occur in the first trimester. The third occurs in the second trimester. Some discrimination probably should be made between the first two months of the third trimester and the 9th month of pregnancy. There is a slight tendency for women with problems about their pregnancy to have an elevation in psychological problems as measured by the CPI during the second trimester. We believe this phenomenon may be related to "quickening." During the last month the effects of psychological and stress factors are believed to be modulated and masked by the physiological strain on the women and the increased secretion of hormones.

Psychologically and on the basis of the indexing of the pregnancy processes, four phases of pregnancy are discriminated by our data: the first trimester, the second trimester, the seventh and eighth months, and the ninth month.

Stress and Pregnancy:

As indicated earlier, the CBY program extended its data set and conceptualization beyond that of the original PIPAS project. The primary addition of variables was that of nutrition and aerobic exercises. All of these variables: demographic, obstetrical history, health history, symptom proneness, CPI, and pregnancy symptoms are related in complex networks, which take different patterns in different women. Generally speaking, stress is a background variable which is a quality of life indicator. The better the quality of life, the lower the stress.

Stress is one of the indicators that affect the abilities of individuals to control their life and to perform the orderly, rational tasks of nutrition, exercise, personal care, and planning and responsibility for optimal health care during pregnancy. The effects of stress are in conjunction with such indices as general symptom proneness (and possibly illness proneness). How all of these sets of variables are related in the CBY conceptual framework is given in Figure 2.

A CBY program goal is to enhance not only the optimal outcomes of the baby, labor, and delivery, but also the quality of pregnancy. In Figure 2, quality of pregnancy is defined in terms of the amount of frequent pregnancy symptoms a woman reports during the first and second trimester. The third trimester symptoms were excluded because of the lower number of cases.

The path diagram of Figure 2 was based upon 32 cases on which data for each variable was complete. It was found that 72% of the symptoms reported during pregnancy were associated with the set of variables. The path diagram is to be read from left to right. The arrows are presumed casual chains between the variables and the special indices.

FIGURE 2 Path Analysis of Selected Variables to Quality of Living Style (Q Living Style) and Quality of Pregnancy**

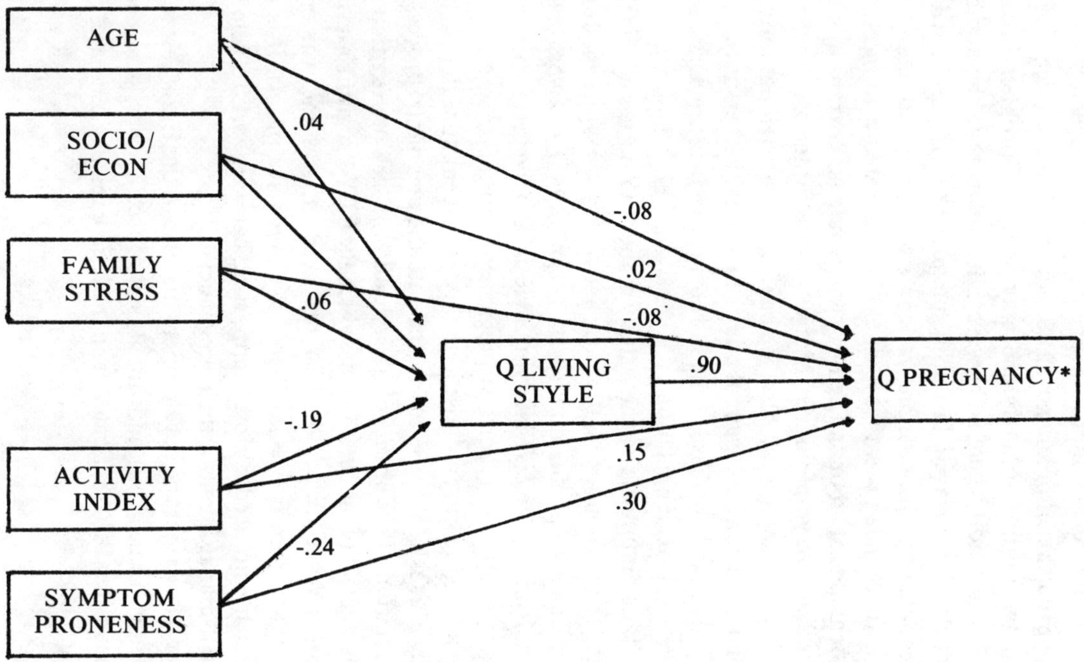

*Corrected R^2 = .71549 which is percent of pregnancy symptoms explained by the set of variables.

**No calculations were made of this set of variables on labor and delivery complications and baby complications because of small numbers of cases. This will be done in the future.

Most interesting is the contribution to pregnancy symptoms of the variable Q Living Style. This index is composed of the CPI scale combined with two stress measures, stresses due to changes in personal habits (Personal Habits Changes Stress) and stresses due to general living patterns (Lifestyle Stress).

In general, as the problems of living style went up so did pregnancy symptoms. Similarly as symptom proneness and aerobic activity went up, so did the problems of pregnancy. The findings about physical activities are a counterintuitive anomaly and may be only a problem in sample variations. The finding here is, however, that increase in the number of physical activities engaged in during pregnancy were associated with more pregnancy symptoms. One rationale for the construction of the physical activity index was that it would be associated with meeting the extreme demands of labor and delivery and would make transition of the ninth month more symptom free. Many exercise enthusiasts learn to live with minor aches and pains. Also, we have not yet sorted out those who have a modest aerobic program of one or two activities versus those with many activities, with increased time and energy expenditure. Data are still being collected on these relations.

The striking finding of this mini-study of the CBY data is how little are the effects of socioeconomic status, age, and family stress on symptoms of pregnancy, and thus the quality of pregnancy. The overwhelming impression from Figure 2 is that living style, as defined in this mini-study, has a strong relation to reports of pregnancy symptoms.

The social engineering of those living styles that enhance the quality of pregnancy is a task for those concerned with the pregnancy process. The underestimation of the effects of lifestyle and the lack of attention to its features is a defect of the care system, which the CBY Program is trying to remedy. It is a striking finding of this study that some women are practically symptom free, but others have many symptoms. It is these latter women who need a close, supporting care network to help their optimal self-management of their pregnancies.

Chapter 4 describes the development and use of the Utah Test for the Childbearing Year. This additional set of scales was designed to complement the PIPAS Scales, and further expands our stress and pregnancy model.

References

Foster, J. (1981). Building a healthy baby: Nutrition for pregnancy. Slide-tape (11 minutes) and instructor's manual. University of Utah Instructional Media Services, Salt Lake City, Utah.

Kitzinger, S. (1977). *Education and counseling for childbirth.* London: Bailliere Tindall.

Selected Bibliography

Cameron, J. (1979). Year-long classes for couples becoming parents. *American Journal of Nursing,* 6, *4,* 358-362.

Cooper, M. & Cooper, K.H. (1972). *Aerobics for women.* New York: Bantam Books (M. Evans & Co. Inc.).

Foster, J. (1981). Building a healthy baby: Nutrition for pregnancy. Slide-tape (11 Minutes) and instructor's manual. University of Utah Instructional Media Services, Salt Lake City, Utah.

Jacobson, E. (1964). *Anxiety and tension control.* Philadelphia: Lippincot.

Kitzinger, S. (1977). *Education and counseling for childbirth.* London: Bailliere Tindall.

Lamaze, F. (1984). *Painless childbirth: The lamaze method.* Chicago: Contemporary Books, Inc.

4
Utah Test For The Childbearing Year

Introduction

Although the PIPAS system of measures was unusually successful in measuring stress, the general weakness was that psychological variables were only roughly indexed by the psychiatric items of the CPI. The psychological stresses of the pregnant woman were only noted in terms of pathological effects, and no indications are given of the contents of the stresses. A woman's beliefs and perceptions about childbearing may also constitute additional stressors affecting the quality and outcome of the pregnancy experience. These beliefs and perceptions may serve as powerful predisposing factors impacting her health care decisions and practices.

What we needed as clinicians caring for the pregnant woman was an assessment of the woman's perceptions and beliefs about such factors as fear of childbearing, childbirth health locus of control, personal values about childbearing and childrearing, passive compliance versus active participation in childbirth care decisions, and the role and responsibility of the father.

The support that the clinician can give to the psychologically stressed pregnant woman depends upon an accurate assessment of these psychological dimensions. For this reason, we moved the research program into the development of an additional battery of scales that were closely associated with the problems the clinician faces in actual practice.

The Utah Test for the Childbearing Year: Beliefs and Perceptions about Childbearing was developed to address the need for a set of valid, reliable scales that could contribute to another aspect of identification of stress/risk factors during pregnancy. We felt that such a set of scales would be useful to childbirth educators and health care providers in identifying the kind and amount of support and education required by specific individuals and groups.

We envisioned the combination of the PIPAS and Beliefs and Perceptions Scales as a next step toward developing a predictive index and providing a prescription for intervention. An understanding of the normative childbearing beliefs and perceptions in any given population would facilitate planning for maternity health care services in a community. We also believed that these scales would be useful to both researchers and clinicians interested in the association of risk variables with various pregnancy outcomes.

Two potential areas of impact for five selected domains of childbearing beliefs and perceptions are presented in Figure 1. It is hypothesized that health *behaviors* have potential for influencing the wellbeing of either or both the mother and the fetus/neonate. The second area of impact is that mediated directly on maternal and/or fetal outcome through *pathophysiological changes* brought on by various stressors, such as the effect of maternal anxiety on premature labor and other labor complications (Crandon, 1978; Erickson, 1976a, 1976b; Lederman, Lederman, Work & McCann, 1978; McDonald, 1968; Myers, 1977; Newton, Webster, Binu, Maskrey, & Phillips, 1979).

Widespread use of public media has made new information available to expectant parents regarding desirable health care behaviors during pregnancy. Nutrition, physical fitness, stress reduction, and avoidance of personal habits hazards and environmental hazards are all topics discussed in popular and scientific literature. The extent to which parents avail themselves of this knowledge may be influenced by their beliefs and perceptions about childbearing and health.

In our western society, the concept of an optimal pregnancy outcome ranges from a minimal expectancy for a live mother and infant without overt physical or mental damage, to an expectation by an increasing number of couples that the process of childbearing should be a satisfying period of increased development as a person, culminating in a peak childbirth experience as well (Tanzer, 1972). Phrases such as "participatory decision making," "family involvement," and "maximal possible control over the birth experience" are appearing in the literature. Individuals who hold these values usually seek additional information

Hypothesized Impact of Beliefs and Perceptions About Childbearing

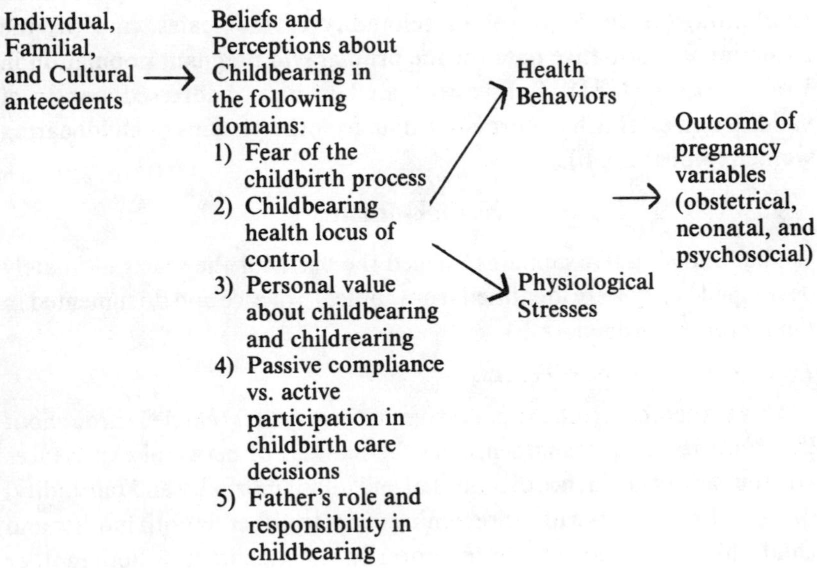

Figure 1.

and skill development to increase their competence and sense of confidence. They are also likely to seek alternative approaches to managing the course of childbearing (Arms, 1975; Haire, 1972; Howell, 1975; Kitzinger, 1962). Difficulty in obtaining these desired experiences can result in various degrees of stress within the expectant couple.

Conversely, other couples believe that a safe and healthy mother and baby is the responsibility of their physician. Those who hold this position tend to believe their responsibility is to select a physician who will see that they experience little or no pain or distress during the birth process. Other individuals' beliefs and practices range within the continuum represented by these extremes (Parlee, 1976; Stewart, 1977; Wheeler, 1977).

Therefore, the Utah Test for the Childbearing Year was designed to identify the stress/wellness continuum along which individuals may be placed, based on their response to statements of belief and perception relative to selected concepts, within specified domains.

The initial study was limited to (a) scale construction, (b) content validation, (c) development of reliability of the scales, and (d) the gathering of normative data for the primigravid pregnant population in Utah (Foster, 1981). Subsequent studies have addressed construct validity and established normative data for other groups of childbearing women (Appendix F).

Scale Domains

The following five domains formed the basis for the scales ultimately developed. They were identified from clinical practice and documented in the literature (Appendix E).

Fear of the Childbirth Process

This fear comes from the pervasive cultural beliefs (carried throughout the centuries, and strengthened by the realities of personal experiences and the varying incidence of maternal and infant mortality and morbidity) that childbirth: (a) is a life-threatening event to either or both mother and child, (b) can permanently or temporarily damage either or both mother and child, (c) is an unpleasant experience, (d) is a frightening experience, (e) is a painful experience.

Psychological stress and maternal attitudes during pregnancy have been found to affect adversely the outcome of pregnancy, labor, and delivery through such problems as premature or dysfunctional labor, neonatal morbidity, etc. (Davids, Devault & Talmadge, 1961; Erickson, 1965). Conversely, positive correlates of these beliefs may also be found, especially since the early 1950's. The childbirth education literature is replete with descriptions of confident, unafraid women during pregnancy and childbirth, who cope successfully with the sensations of labor (Dick-Read, 1944; Kitzinger, 1962, Lamaze, 1970; Tanzer, 1972).

Childbearing Health Locus of Control

This domain resulted from the application of the individual difference construct, internal-external locus of control, from Rotter's social learning theory (Rotter, 1954; Rotter, Chance & Phares, 1972) to the area of health care, with specific focus on childbearing. "The internal-external dimension pertains to a person's expectancy that his/her reinforcements are under either personal (termed internal) or environmental (termed external control" (Stokols, 1975, p. 135.). Childbearing-specific items relate to the three multidimensional aspects of locus of control (as identified by Wallston, Kaplan, and Maides (1976); Wallston, Maides, and Wallston (1976); and Wallston and Wallston (1976) in their Multidimensional Health Locus of Control Scales): (a) Internality, (b) Powerful Others (externality), (c) Fate or Chance (externality).

Childbearing-specific dimensions of the domain include (a) information seeking regarding childbearing and health care, (b) taking preventive measures to maximize health care practices, (c) responses to options and choices in childbirth health care practices, (d) responses to medical authority, and (e) belief in personal ability to bear a child safely and successfully (i.e., personal health, normalcy, strength, and willingness to participate in and work with the process of labor).

Personal Values About Childbearing and Childrearing

Today there is a wide range of values placed on bearing a child and becoming a parent, from a decision never to become pregnant to yearning for that opportunity on the part of infertile couples. Some individuals feel that the pregnancy process enhances their self-development and self-fulfillment as a person. The process is seen variously, ranging from one to be endured to one to be welcomed as a positive human experience. The child is viewed on a continuum from a burden imposed on self and society to fulfillment of one's ultimate reason for being. Lifestyle changes are perceived as minimal to profound with negative, neutral, or positive feelings regarding these changes. Commitment to an optimal outcome ranges from letting pregnancy take its course, through specific actions if they are easy and do not require much energy or change, to willingness to exert maximum energy and effort. The dimensions identified in the literature included (a) desire to produce a child of one's own (b) belief in pregnancy, childbirth, and parenting as a personal growth-producing experience, (c) basic meaning of producing a child, (d) perceived effect on one's lifestyle, and (e) commitment to working for an optimal outcome.

The perceived relationship between pregnancy, childbirth, and parenting and one's personal self-development and self-fulfillment is identified by items measuring: (a) desire to be a parent, (b) personal meaning and value of childbearing and childrearing, (c) enjoyment of babies and children, (d) perceived effect of children on a marriage, (e) perceived risks and responsibilities of parenting.

Passive Compliance versus Active Participation in Childbirth Care Decisions

The individual's beliefs are located along a continuum of beliefs from passive compliance with the childbirth care system to a mutually interactive process utilizing one's own resources as well as those within the system. The beliefs that enter into this domain concern the necessity/desirability for essentially unquestioning compliance with the professionals' and the systems' usual approaches to childbirth care versus a belief that there are a number of different but equally safe ways to approach childbirth, and a desire to participate in decisions and use one's own resources maximally. This domain might also be characterized as dependence versus interdependence with health care providers and the health care system.

Father's Role and Response in Childbearing

The effects of childbirth on the father, and of the father on the childbirth experience of the mother are described in numerous articles in the literature (Chiota, Goolkasian, & Ladewig, 1976; Cobb, 1976; Fawcett, 1978; Henneborn & Cogan, 1975; Hollender & McGehee, 1974; Peterson, Mehl, & Leiderman, 1979; Pies, Reid, 1975; Trethowan & Conlon, 1965; Wilson, 1970). Responses range from ignoring the partner to extreme dependence. There is a range of beliefs about both the desire, ability, and right of the father to be involved in childbearing and parenting, and also the woman's need and desire for his involvement. The perceived paternal role and responses are measured by items identifying: (a) the desirability of father involvement, support, agreement, and congruence with his partner; (b) the need for and importance of father involvement, support, agreement, and congruence with his partner; (c) the perceived ability of the father to become involved, be supportive, agree, and be in congruence with his partner; (d) the perceived ability of the mother to function successfully in the physical absence of the father and/or the absence of his involvement, support, agreement, and/or congruence.

Methodology

Development of the scales followed procedures for measurement of sentiments according to established psychometric theory as described by Nunnally (1978). The final product is a five-scale paper and pencil test, appropriate for both men and women during their years of reproductive capacity. The scores obtained with the instrument can be used, among other possibilities, in correlation studies with pregnancy symptoms, selected health behaviors during childbearing, and pregnancy outcomes. The scales may also be used to determine changeability of scores and behaviors through the influence of childbirth health education programs, thus providing another source of input for program evaluation.

Step one in the development of the scales involved the general conceptualization of the domains described above. Steps two through nine involved: (Step 2) review of the literature, (3) development of an item pool, (4) submission of the original item pool to an expert panel, (5) pretest of selected items, (6) preparation of the final edition of the initial instrument, (7) initial administration of the instrument to establish reliability of the items, (8) analysis of items administered to the general population, and (9) administration of the revised instrument to a representative sample of 254 pregnant primigravid women and 253 of their partners (Foster, 1981).

Results

Demographic Data:

The expectant fathers averaged about 25 years of age while the expectant mothers were about 23 years old. Ages ranged from 15 to 38 years. All but a very few of the couples were married Caucasians. Average family income was approximately $18,000 with a standard deviation of about $12,000. A set of 11 categories of occupations were derived by John Sullivan from the Department of Labor Occupational Classifications. All 11 of the occupational groups were represented, with approximately 32% of the men reporting that they were professionals (including college students). The next most commonly reported occupations (approximately 13% each) were proprietor or manager of a business and craftsman. The 3 most common occupational groups reported by the women were clerical (28%), homemaker (25%), and professional (22%, included college students). (Table 1.)

Compared with the general population group in the initial study, the expectant couples were 4-6 years younger, made an average of $4,000 a year less, were almost all married, had no children currently, and an average of two years less education. There was a smaller number reporting a professional/college student occupation. They were similar in racial background.

FORTAP Analysis of the Domain Scales:

The Alpha coefficients for the primigravid women ranged from .63 to .76; those of the first-time expectant fathers ranged from .63 to .78 (Table 2). Reliability of the scale Fear of the Childbirth Process was higher for the primigravid women than the men (.76 versus .68). Reliability of the scale Father's Role and Responses in Childbearing and Childrearing was higher for the first-time expectant fathers than for the primigravid women (.72 versus .65). Also the reliability for the scale Childbearing Health Locus of Control was greater for the women than for the men (.71 versus .66). There was little or no difference in reliability scores between men and women on the scales Personal Values About Childbearing and Childrearing (.78 vs. .76), and Passive Compliance versus Active Participation in Childbirth Care Decisions (both .63).

Compared to their partners, the women reported slightly less fear of the childbirth process, a slightly higher internal locus of control, personal value regarding childrearing and childbearing, and belief in the father's role and responses in childbearing and childrearing. They perceived themselves as only slightly more likely to be passively compliant versus actively participating in childbirth-care decisions, compared to their partners.

Compared to the expectant couples, the general population (nonpregnant) reported comparatively less fear of the childbirth process, had a higher internal locus of control, a much lower personal value about childbearing and childrearing, valued the father's role and responses in

TABLE 1
Demographic Data

Data	Salt Lake and Weber Counties General Population Sample N=382 Subjects Reporting					Utah Pregnant Primigravidas N=254 Subjects Reporting				
	Number	Percent	Range	Mean	SD	Number	Percent	Range	Mean	SD
Sex:	350	92				254	100			
Males	99	26				—	—			
Females	251	66				254	100			
Age (years)	346	91	15-59	28.9	8.6	254	100	15-35	22.6	3.4
Marital Status:	352	92				254	100			
Single	136	36				6	2.4			
Married	179	47				248	97.6			
Windowed	2	.5				—	—			
Separated	2	.5				—	—			
Divorced	33	8.6				—	—			
Race:	351	92				253	99.6			
Caucasian	300	86				246	97.2			
Black	6	1.6				—	—			
Asian	6	1.3				—	—			
American Indian	1	.3				2	.8			
Hispanic	9	2.4				4	1.6			
Number of Children	352	92	0-8	1.3	1.8	254	100	0	—	—

TABLE 1 *(continued)*

Demographic Data

	Salt Lake and Weber Counties General Population Sample N=382					Utah Pregnant Primigravidas N=254				
	Subjects Reporting					Subjects Reporting				
Data	Number	Percent	Range	Mean	SD	Number	Percent	Range	Mean	SD
Total Family Income/Year	298	78	0-$100,000	$21,797	$15,305	225	88.6	$3,000-$99,000	$17,972.27	$11,478.18
Years of Education	351	92	9-20	15	2	253	99.6	8-26	13.72	1.98
Occupation:	332	87				253	99.6			
Professional including student	217	57				57	22.4			
Clerical	33	8.6				72	28.3			
Homemaker	26	6.8				64	25.2			
Other Service Worker	19	5				19	7.5			
Prop. or Mgr. of Business or Agriculture	11	2.9				7	2.8			
Domestic Worker	8	2				4	1.6			
High School/Trade School Student	7	1.8				5	2.0			
Operator	4	1.0				9	3.5			
Craftsman	2	.5				2	.8			
Salesman	2	.5				11	4.3			
Laborer/Farm Worker	0	0				3	1.2			

FORTAP Analysis of Final Instrument Data

Domain	Number of Items	Mother Data - N=254: N of Items[a] Answered in Scored Direction: Mean	S.D.	Alpha Coefficient	Father Data - N=253: N of Items[a] Answered in Scored Direction: Mean	S.D.	Alpha Coefficient
Fear of the Child-birth Process	21	9.97	4.11	.76	10.74	3.65	.68
Childbearing Health Locus of Control	20	6.32	3.17	.71	7.21	3.09	.66
Personal Values About Childbearing and Childrearing	15	3.56	2.88	.76	3.66	3.00	.78
Father's Role and Response in Child-bearing and Childrearing	24	3.70	2.73	.65	4.62	3.23	.72
Passive Compliance vs. Active Participation in Childbirth Care Decisions	20	6.07	2.60	.63	6.36	2.78	.63
Total Number of Items	100	—	—	—	—	—	—

[a]The scored direction is toward the negative, i.e., fear of childbirth, high externality, low value, low role, and passive compliance.

childbearing and childrearing less, and were more likely to believe in passive compliance rather than active participation in childbirth-care decisions.

Factor Analysis of the Domain Scales

We next factor analyzed the five domain scales to test for the independence of the domains. Initially, the most widely used factor analysis was run in which, for the Statistical Package for the Social Sciences (SPSS) system, all of the default options were taken: principal axis with iteration and a varimax rotation with an Eigenvalue of 1. There were two factors that together explained 69.9% of the variance of the scales. The first factor accounted for 45.6% of the variance of the scales, and the second factor accounted for 24.4% of the variance. In this particular analysis the Father's Role and Response in Childbearing scale was not highly loaded on either factor.

The first factor had an underlying dimension of which each of the three scales (Fear of the Childbirth Process, Combined Childbearing Health Locus of Control, and Passive Compliance versus Active Participation in Childbirth Care Decisions) is a manifestation. This dimension has been labeled Childbearing Self-Competency. There was a Combined Childbearing Health Locus of Control loading of .86112, a Passive Compliance versus Active Participation with Childbirth Care Decisions loading of .85859, and a Fear of the Childbirth Process loading of .60581.

The second factor had as a high loading the Personal Values About Childbearing and Childrearing scale at .69074. This Personal Values About Childbearing and Childrearing scale was slightly negatively loaded (-.12894) on factor one.

The second analysis performed was similar to the first with the exception that the sub-scale Childbearing Health Locus of Control — Powerful Others was substituted for the combined Locus of Control scale. Our rationale for this substitution was that it made the analysis closer to the clinical situation in which the health care providers are frequently seen as powerful by pregnant women. This analysis also took the default options of the SPSS and was the basis of the circumplex model described below.

A third factor analysis was run in which the parameters were a principal component analysis with an oblique rotation controlled by a delta = -.5. The minimum Eigenvalue was .65 and was determined by the high intercorrelation of the scales. In this analysis, three factors were identified accounting for 83.3% of the variance of the scales. The first factor, which had an Eigenvalue of 2.15802 and accounted for 42.3% of the variance, had the following as factor loadings: Passive Compliance versus Active Participation in Childbirth Care Decisions = .99035, Childbearing Health Locus of Control — Powerful Others = .55988, and Fear of the Childbirth Process = .46024. Thus, this factor is almost a pure measure of Passive Compliance versus Active Participation in Childbirth Care Decisions. The second factor, with an Eigenvalue of 1.24568 accounting for 24.9% of the variance, was Personal Values About Childbearing and Childrearing and is almost a pure measure with a loading of .99880. The third factor had a Eigenvalue of .78804 and accounted for 15.8% of the variance of the five scales. It was negatively loaded and is almost a pure measure of Father's Role and Response in Childbearing.

Circumplex Model

The circumplex model (Figure 2) was constructed from a principal axis factoring with a varimax rotation. This rotation results in the factors being orthogonal to each other which fits the requirements of having the axes of the circumplex model perpendicular to each other. Each individual factor score for Personal Values About Childbearing and Childrearing and Childbearing Self-Competency was computed and plotted on the two dimensional grid.

Childbearing Self-Competency, you will recall, consists of the three scales: (a) Fear of the Childbirth Process, (b) Childbearing Health Locus of Control — Powerful Others, and (c) Passive Compliance versus Active Participation in Childbirth Care Decisions. The 49 items in this construct, and the 15 items in the Personal Values scale resulted in a total of 64 items necessary for the circumplex model.

The average standard deviation of the two factors was computed, and a circle drawn whose radius was one standard deviation. A second circle delineated two standard deviations. As a result of these plots we identified

FIGURE 2

Utah Primagravidas N = 254

Personal Values About Childbearing and Childrearing

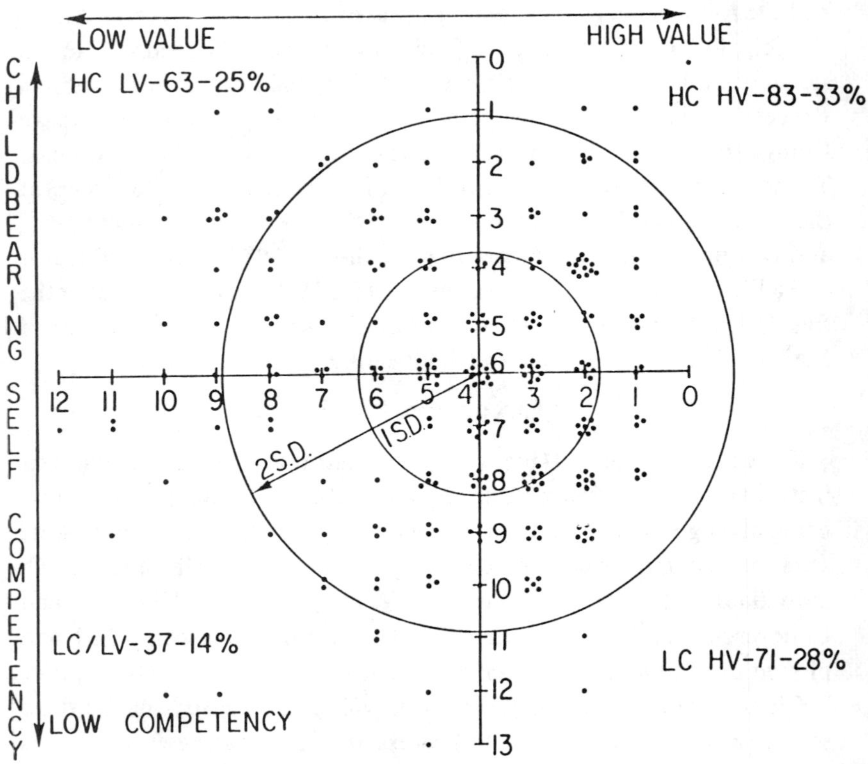

the following four groups of individuals in the Utah primivigrad population: (a) High Childbearing Self Competency and High Values About Childbearing and Childrearing — 33%, (b) High Childbearing Self-Competency and Low Values About Childbearing and Childrearing — 25%, (c) Low Childbearing Self-Competency and High Values About Childbearing and Childrearing — 28%, and (d) Low Childbearing Self-Competency and Low Values About Childbearing and Childrearing —14%.

The four groups are presented in descending order of presumed risk and need for intervention. The relationship, if any, between these individuals in each of the four groups and process or outcome of pregnancy, is still to be determined through future research. We believe that this grid has potential use for plotting and comparing individual/couple responses to the scales. It could also be used to plot change within individuals over time as a result of interventions such as prenatal classes, individual counseling, etc.

Individual Profile Sheet

Finally we prepared an individual profile sheet (Figure 3). We placed the number of items in each scale according to the mean and standard deviation for that scale. This permits the number of items in the scored direction for an individual, from each of the five major domain scales and the three sub-groups of the Childbearing Health Locus of Control scale to be visually compared with the normative data for the 254 Utah Primigravid Women.

An individual with a score or scores greater than one standard deviation might need further evaluation and, depending on the scale, intervention. For example, an extremely fearful individual might benefit from the support and information available from a series of classes in childbirth preparation. In the examples used in Figure 3 two different women from the present study are represented by their scale scores. As can readily be seen, one is essentially low-risk, while the other is high-risk, according to the hypothesized model.

We have found these profiles to be extremely useful to the childbirth educator/health professional in more sensitively gearing his/her

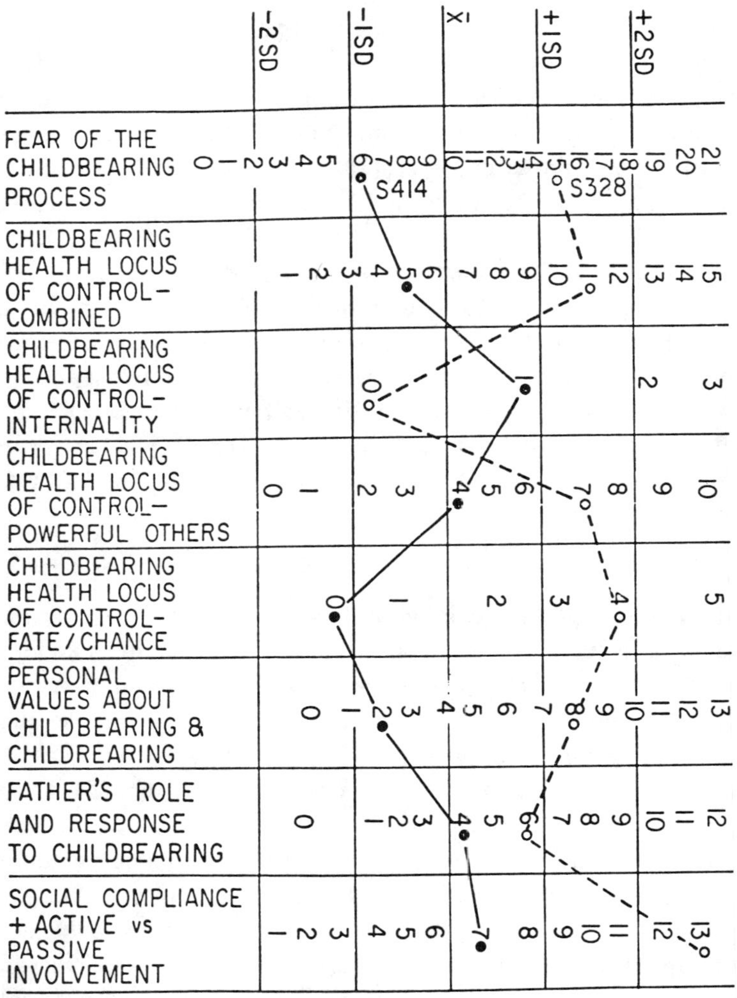
+2SD
+1SD
x̄
-1SD
-2SD
FEAR OF THE CHILDBEARING PROCESS
S414
S328
CHILDBEARING HEALTH LOCUS OF CONTROL-COMBINED
CHILDBEARING HEALTH LOCUS OF CONTROL-INTERNALITY
CHILDBEARING HEALTH LOCUS OF CONTROL-POWERFUL OTHERS
CHILDBEARING HEALTH LOCUS OF CONTROL-FATE/CHANCE
PERSONAL VALUES ABOUT CHILDBEARING & CHILDREARING
FATHER'S ROLE AND RESPONSE TO CHILDBEARING
SOCIAL COMPLIANCE + ACTIVE vs PASSIVE INVOLVEMENT

FIGURE 3

program/care toward individual and group needs. We see this profile sheet as an addition to the PIPAS profile sheet.

The next five sections describe the normative data in each of the five domains. Frequencies, and correlations of total scale scores with the demographic, health behavioral, and childbearing data will be presented.

Normative Data: Fear of the Childbirth Process:

The women responded with a mean of 9.97 of the 21 items in the scored direction, i.e. indicating fear. With a standard deviation of 4.11 items, two-thirds of the group rated between 6 and 14 items in the direction of fear of the childbirth process. The variability in response makes this scale a sensitive indicator of fear. The response to individual items in this scale is presented in Table 1, Appendix E.

Younger and less educated women were the most fearful. The more fearful women used significantly fewer stress reduction activities and made significantly greater use of car safety belts. They also had less confidence in their ability to cope with the labor and delivery process, and they had read significantly fewer books on childbirth and parenting. Correlations between fear and the other domain scales indicated that fearful women are more likely to be externally directed and passively compliant in relation to their childbirth experience (Table 3).

Normative Data: Childbearing Health Locus of Control

There are 20 items in this combined scale, with the three subsets (scales) of this domain: Internality — 6 items, Externality-Powerful Others — 8 items, and Externality-Fate/Chance — 6 items. For the combined scale the women responded with a mean of 6.32 items in the scored direction, i.e., toward externality, indicating that they were more internally oriented as a group than externally oriented. With a standard deviation of 3.17 items, two-thirds of the group rated between 3 and 9 items of the total 20 items in the direction of external locus of control. Most of the women believed in the importance of personal health practices as the best means of influencing the outcome of pregnancy, and that they could have the kind of childbearing experience they want, and have an easier childbirth through their own efforts (Table 2, Appendix E).

Pearson Product Moment Correlations for this domain indicated significant negative correlations with 13 other variables. As externality increased the following decreased: age, total family income, education, number of abortions/miscarriages, percent attendance at scheduled prenatal classes, confidence to cope with labor and delivery, number of childbirth and parenting books read, practice of breathing and relaxation exercises, use of aerobic exercise and stress reduction activities, and the number of days in seven a nutritious diet was eaten. Externally oriented women made greater use of physician health care providers and reported less personal values about childbearing and childrearing.

There were nine variables with significant positive correlations with externality. Externally oriented women made greater use of car safety belts, but began prenatal care later in their pregnancy and were more likely to use traditional sites for delivery. They evidenced both greater fear of the childbirth process, and dependence on powerful others or fate/chance. They were more passively compliant and minimized the father's role and response.

A mean of 4.22 in the scored direction, i.e., toward reliance on powerful others, of the eight items representing this scale, indicates that the group was divided in their orientation toward powerful others. The standard deviation of 2.27 items indicated that two-thirds of the group rated between two and six items in the direction of powerful others. The variance indicates that this is a sensitive indicator of orientation toward powerful others in relation to childbearing. In this population half or more of the women agreed with following the health providers advice without question, going along with his/her usual practices in labor and delivery, and believed just being in the hospital would make them feel safe. However, only 28% believed they should do what they are told regardless of personal preference, and only 36% agreed that it was best to leave decisions about maternity care to the professionals.

In this population, the group as a whole did not hold beliefs relative to fate or chance. There was a mean of 1.58 in the scored direction, i.e., toward belief in fate or chance, of the six items in this scale. A standard deviation of 1.21 items meant that two-thirds of the group rated between zero and three items in the scored direction (Tables 4,5,6,7).

TABLE 3

Correlation of Demographic, Health Behavior, and Childbearing Variables and Domain Scores with the Domain: Fear of the Childbirth Process

Variable Group	Number of Subjects Reporting	Pearson Correlation	Significance Level P Value
Demographic Data:			
Age	254	-.1586	.001
Educational Level	253	-.1221	.052
Health Behavior Data:			
Stress Reduction/7 Days	250	-.1860	.003
Use of Car Safety Belt	254	.1782	.004
Childbearing Data:			
Confidence to Cope with Labor and Delivery	243	-.3632	.001
Ease of Pregnancy	253	.1227	.051
Number of Childbirth/Parenting Books Read	249	-.1527	.016
Breathing/Relaxation/7 Days	251	-.1493	.018
Domain Scale Scores:			
Combined Childbearing Locus of Control	254	.5259	.001
Childbearing Locus of Control—Powerful Others	254	.2171	.001
Childbearing Locus of Control—Fate/Chance	254	.4325	.001
Passive Compliance vs. Active Participation in Childbirth Care Decisions	254	.5415	.001

Normative Data: Personal Values About Childbearing

There was a mean response of 3.56 items n the scored direction, i.e., toward minimal value, out of the 15 possible items in this domain. With a standard deviation of 2.88 items, two-thirds of the group placed between 0 and 6 items in the scored direction, indicating a high value for childbearing and childrearing by this population (Table 3, Appendix E).

Increased value of childbearing is significantly positively correlated with increased age, education, and income. Women with an increased number of previous miscarriages reflect that the present pregnancy is highly valued, probably because of previous failed attempts at childbearing. Increased value is also correlated with greater internality, less dependance on powerful others, and an increased sense of the importance of the father's role and response to childbearing. Two unexplained correlations with this scale, which may be spurious, are decreased use of car safety belts and increased number of cigarettes smoked in 24 hours (Table 8).

Normative Data: Father's Role and Response in Childbearing

There is great importance placed on the father's role and response in this population. There was a mean response of 2.71 items in the scored direction, i.e., toward minimal role and response, out of 24 total items in this scale. The standard deviation was 2.73 items, therefore two-thirds of the group rated between 1 and 6 items in the scored direction. Ten items relating to the need and desirability for the husband's support and sustaining presence throughout pregnancy and childbirth were supported by 67 to 99% of the study population. Over 80% of the respondents believed that expectant fathers also have increased needs during pregnancy and a lot of fears and concerns. Only 24% believed that pregnancy is not physically stressful for an expectant father (Table 4, Appendix E).

The Father's Role and Response Scale had a significant positive correlation with all of the other domain scales except personal value of childbearing and childrearing. There was no relationship between value of childbearing per se and value of the father's role and response in childbearing. As the father's role was minimized there was a concomitant increase in fear, externality, and passive compliance. Younger women

TABLE 4

Correlation of Demographic, Health Behavior, and Childbearing Variables and Domain Scores with the Domain: Childbearing Health Locus of Control — Combined

Variable Group	Number of Subjects Reporting	Pearson Correlation	Significance Level P Value
Demographic Data:			
Age	254	-.3377	.001
Total Family Income	225	.1503	.024
Education Level	253	.3005	.001
Health Behavior Data:			
Aerobic Exercise/7 Days	253	-.2163	.001
Stress Reduction/7 Days	250	-.2296	.001
Nutritious Diet/7 Days	254	-.2599	.011
Use of Car Safety Belt	254	.2791	.001
Childbearing Data:			
Number of Abortions	254	-.1480	.018
Attendance at Scheduled Prenatal classes	86	-.2094	.053
Confidence to Cope with Labor and Delivery	243	-.338	.001
Month Prenatal Care Began	253	.1448	.021
Number of Childbirth/ Parenting Books Read	249	-.2027	.001
Breathing/Relaxation/7 Days	251	-.2577	.001
Planned Delivery Site	252	.3082	.001
Health Care Provider	253	-.1546	.014

TABLE 4 *Continued*

Variable Group	Number of Subjects Reporting	Pearson Correlation	Significance Level P Value
Domain Scale Scores:			
Fear of the Childbirth Process	254	.5259	.001
Personal Values About Childbearing and Childrearing	254	-.1265	.044
Childbearing Health Locus of Control — Internality	254	.4169	.001
Childbearing Health Locus of Control — Powerful Others	254	.8902	.001
Childbearing Health Locus of Control — Fate/Chance	254	.6605	.001
Father's Role and Response	254	.2365	.001
Passive Compliance vs. Active Participation in Childbirth Care Decisions	254	.7226	.001

with one or no miscarriages were significantly correlated with minimizing the father's role and response (Table 9).

Normative Data: Passive Compliance versus Active Participation in Childbirth Care Decisions

There are 20 items in this scale with a mean response of 6.07 items in the scored direction, i.e., toward passive compliance. The standard deviation of 2.60 items, indicated that two-thirds of the group rated between 3 and 9 items in the scored direction and believed in more active participation in childbirth care decisions. Responses to particular beliefs, represented by individual items in this domain, are seen in Table 5, Appendix E.

As passive compliance increases, the following are significantly decreased: age, educational level, number of abortions/miscarriages, use of aerobic exercise, stress reduction activities, eating a nutritious diet, confidence to cope with labor and delivery, weeks gestation, number of books read, and practice of breathing and relaxation exercises. Passive

TABLE 5

Correlation of Demographic, Health Behavior, and Childbearing Variables and Domain Scores with the Domain: Childbearing Health Locus of Control — Internally

Variable Group	Number of Subjects Reporting	Pearson Correlation	Significance Level P Value
Demographic Data:			
Total Family Income	225	-.1430	.032
Health Behavior Data:			
Aerobic Exercise/7 Days	253	-.1312	.037
Stress Reduction/7 Days	250	-.1760	.005
Childbearing Data:			
Attendance at Scheduled Prenatal Classes	86	-.3318	.002
Domain Scale Scores:			
Fear of the Childbirth Process	254	.2127	.001
Childbearing Health Locus of Control — Combined	254	.4169	.001
Childbearing Health Locus of Control — Powerful Others	254	.1665	.008
Father's Role and Response	254	.1665	.008
Passive Compliance vs. Active Participation in Childbirth Care Decisions	254	.2802	.001

TABLE 6

Correlation of Demographic, Health Behavior, and Childbearing Variables and Domain Scores with the Domain: Childbearing Health Locus of Control — Powerful Others

Variable Group	Number of Subjects Reporting	Pearson Correlation	Significance Level P Value
Demographic Data:			
Age	254	-.3182	.001
Education Level	253	-.2878	.001
Health Behavior Data:			
Aerobic Exercise/7 Days	253	-.1649	.009
Stress Reduction/7 Days	250	-.2059	.001
Nutritious Diet/7 Days	254	-.1362	.030
Use of Car Safety Belt	254	.2970	.001
Childbearing Data:			
Confidence to Cope with Labor and Delivery	243	-.1976	.002
Number of Abortions	254	-.1726	.006
Number of Childbirth/ Parenting Books Read	249	-.2038	.001
Breathing/Relaxation/7 Days	251	-.2673	.001
Planned Delivery Site	252	.0321	.001
Health Care Provider	253	-.1860	.003
Domain Scales:			
Fear of the Childbirth Process	254	.4253	.001
Personal Values About Childbearing and Childrearing	254	-.2260	.001
Childbearing Health Locus of Control — Combined	254	-.8902	.001
Childbearing Health Locus of Control — Internality	254	.1525	.015
Childbearing Health Locus of Control — Fate/Chance	254	.3497	.001
Father's Role and Response	254	.1511	.016
Passive Compliance vs. Active Participation in Childbirth Care Decisions	254	.6496	.001

compliance is significantly correlated with increased compliance in taking prescribed drugs, use of a car safety belt, later registration for prenatal care, use of more traditional delivery sites, and increased fear of the childbirth process (Table 10).

Summary of the Scales:

For the female group, three of the five scales have adequate reliabilities of .71 to .76 alpha coefficients. The other two (Father's Role and Passive Compliance) have borderline alpha coefficients, .66 and .63, respectively. For the male group, Personal Values and Father's Role have adequate reliability (alpha coefficients .78 and .72) whereas the other three scales have borderline reliability (alpha coefficients .63-.68).

Factor analysis revealed two particularly powerful factors among the five scales: Childbearing Self-Competency and Personal Values About Childbearing and Childrearing. These factors were utilized to create a circumplex model in which individuals' factor scores could be plotted. In addition an individual score profile is possible.

The correlation of scale scores with demographic, health behavior, and childbearing variables was significant and clinically relevant giving some additional evidence of validity. The scales appear to be sensitive enough to make useful distinctions among individuals on the several domains for both practice and research purposes.

We have included the scales in the packet given to the expectant couples in the childbearing year program during the past four years. Because we were expanding the size of the questionnaire, we decided to eliminate the CPI items. We had used CPI data for research purposes but had not shared that information with the couples because we were uncertain how to use it within the confines of an educational program.

The couples have responded very positively to the new profile and the discussions regarding possible implications for health and quality of pregnancy experience. We feel that we are now ready to launch a final project to test an almost complete model. That model and our projections for next steps are discussed in Chapter 5: Summary.

TABLE 7

Correlation of Demographic, Health Behavior, and Childbearing Variables and Domain Scores with the Domain: Childbearing Health Locus of Control — Fate/Chance

Variable Group	Number of Subjects Reporting	Pearson Correlation	Significance Level P Value
Demographic Data:			
Age	254	-.2363	.001
Education Level	253	-.2710	.001
Health Behavior Data:			
Number of Cigarettes/24 hrs.	254	.1414	.024
Aerobic Exercise/7 Days	253	-.1667	.008
Nutritious Diet/7 Days	254	-.1659	.008
Use of Car Safety Belt	254	.1615	.010
Childbearing Data:			
Confidence to Cope with Labor and Delivery	243	-.1623	.011
Month Prenatal Care Began	253	-.1795	.004
Planned Delivery Site	252	.1613	.010
Known Medical and Pregnancy Complications	251	.1246	.079
Domain Scale Scores:			
Fear of the Childbirth Process	254	.4325	.001
Childbearing Health Locus of Control — Combined	254	.6605	.001
Childbearing Health Locus of Control — Powerful Others	254	.3497	.001
Father's Role and Response	254	.2208	.001
Passive Compliance vs. Active Participation in Childbirth Care Decisions	254	.4798	.001

TABLE 8

Correlation of Demographic, Health Behavior, and Childbearing Variables and Domain Scores with the Domain: Personal Values About Childbearing and Childrearing

Variable Group	Number Subjects Reporting	Pearson Correlation	Significance Level P Value
Demographic Data:			
Age	254	.3010	.001
Education Level	253	.1978	.002
Total Family Income	225	.3480	.001
Health Behavior Data:			
Number of Cigarettes/7 Days	254	.1594	.011
Use of Car Safety Belt	254	-.1216	.053
Childbearing Data:			
Number of Abortions	254	.1776	.005
Breathing/Relaxation/7 Days	251	.2051	.001
Domain Scale Scores:			
Childbearing Health Locus of Control — Combined	254	-.1265	.004
Childbearing Health Locus of Control — Powerful Others	254	-.2260	.001
Father's Role and Response	254	.2302	.001

TABLE 9

Correlation of Demographic, Health Behavior, and Childbearing Variables and Domain Scores with the Domain: Father's Role and Response in Childbearing

Variable Group	Number of Subjects Reporting	Pearson Correlation	Significance Level P Value
Demographic Data:			
Age	254	-.1618	.010
Health Behavior Data:			
Over-the-Counter Drugs/7 Days	254	.1459	.020
Use of Car Safety Belt	254	.1318	.036
Childbearing Data:			
Number of Abortions	254	-.1451	.021
Breathing/Relaxation/7 Days	251	-.1384	.028
Planned Delivery Site	252	.1262	.045
Domain Scale Data:			
Fear of the Childbirth Process	254	.2302	.001
Childbearing Health Locus of Control — Combined	254	.2365	.001
Childbearing Health Locus of Control — Internality	254	.1665	.008
Childbearing Health Locus of Control — Powerful Others	254	.1511	.016
Childbearing Health Locus of Control — Fate/Chance	254	.2208	.001
Passive Compliance vs. Active Participation in Childbirth Care Decisions	254	.1972	.002

TABLE 10

Correlation of Demographic, Health Behavior, and Childbearing Variables and Domain Scores with the Domain: Social Compliance and Active vs. Passive Involvement

Variable Group	Number of Subjects Reporting	Pearson Correlation	Significance Level P Value
Demographic Data:			
Age	254	-.1873	.003
Education Level	253	-.1488	.018
Health Behavior Data:			
Breath/Relaxation/7 Days	253	.1249	.047
Aerobic Exercise/7 Days	253	-.1726	.006
Stress Reduction/7 Days	250	-.2638	.001
Nutritious Diet/7 Days	254	-.1218	.053
Use of Safety Belt	254	.2086	.001
Childbearing Data:			
Number of Abortions	254	-.1828	.003
Confidence to Cope with Labor and Delivery	253	-.3736	.001
Weeks Gestation	254	-.1254	.046
Month Prenatal Care Began	253	.1403	.026
Number of Childbirth/ Childbirth/Parenting Books Read	249	-.1535	.015
Breathing/Relaxation/7 Days	251	.2565	.001
Planned Delivery Site	252	.2565	.001
Domain Scale Scores:			
Fear of the Childbirth Process	254	.5415	.001

References

Arms, S. (1975). *Immaculate deception.* Boston: Houghton Mifflin Company.

Chiota, B.J., Goolkasian, P., & Ladewig, P. (1976, January/February). Effects of separation from spouse in pregnancy, labor and delivery, and the postpartum period. *Journal of Obstetric-Gynecologic Nursing,* 21-23.

Crandon, A.J. (1978). Maternal anxiety and obstetric complications. *Journal of Psychosomatic Research, 23,* 109-111.

Davids, A., Devault, S., & Talmadge, M. (1961). Anxiety, pregnancy and childbirth abnormalities. *Journal of Consulting Psychology, 25,* 74-77.

Dick-Read, G. (1944). *Childbirth without fear.* New York: Harper and Row.

Erickson, M.D. (1965). Relationships between psychological attitudes during pregnancy and complications of pregnancy, labor and delivery. Summary. *Proceedings of the 73rd Annual Convention of the American Psychological Association, 1,* 213-214.

Erickson, M.T. (1976b). The relationship between psychological variables and specific complications of pregnancy, labor and delivery. *Journal of Psychosomatic Research, 20,* 207-210.

Fawcett, J. (1978, July/August). Body image and the pregnant couple. *Maternal Child Nursing,* 227-232.

Foster, Joyce Cameron (1981). Utah test for the childbearing year: Beliefs and perceptions about childbearing. Dissertation. University of Utah.

Haire, D. (1972). *The cultural warping of childbirth.* Hillside, N.J.: International Childbirth Education Association.

Henneborn, W.J. & Cogan, R. (1975). The effect of husband participation on reported pain and probability of medication during labor and birth. *Journal of Psychosomatic Research, 19,* 215-222.

Hollender, M.H. & McGehee, J.B. (1974). The wish to be held during pregnancy. *Journal of Psychosomatic Research, 18,* 193-197.

Howell, M.C. (1975). *Helping ourselves: Families and the human networks.* Boston: Beacon Press.

Kitzinger, S. (1962). *The experience of childbirth.* New York: Taplinger Publishing Company, Inc.

Lamaze, F. (1970). *Painless childbirth.* Chicago: Henry Regnery Company.

Lederman, R.P., Lederman, E., Work, B.A., & McCann, D.S. (1978). The relationship of maternal anxiety, plasma catacholamines and plasma cortisol to progress labor. *American Journal of Obstetrics and Gynecology, 132,* 5, 495-499.

McDonald, R.L. (1968). The role of emotional factors in obstetric complications: A review. *Psychosomatic Medicine, 30,* 2, 222-234.

Myers, R.E. (1977). Production of fetal asphyxia by maternal psychological stress. *Pavlovian Journal of Biological Science, 12,* 1, 51-61.

Newton, R.W., Webster, P.A.C., Binu, P.S., Maskrey, N., & Phillips, A.B. (1979). Psychosocial stress in pregnancy and its relation to the onset of premature labor. *British Medical Journal, 2,* 411-413.

Nunnally, J.C. (1978). *Psychometric methods.* New York: McGraw-Hill.

Parlee, M.M. (1976). Social factors in the psychology of menstruation, birth and menopause. *Primary Care, 3,* 3, 477-488.

Peterson, G.H., Mehl, L.E., & Leiderman, H.P. (1979). The role of some birth-related variables in father attachment. *American Journal of Orthopsychiatry, 49,* 2, 330-338.

Pies, H.E. (1976). The right of a father to be present in the delivery room. *American Journal of Public Health, 66,* 7, 688-689.

Reid, K.E. (1975, Spring). Fatherhood and emotional stress: The couvade syndrome. *Journal of Social Welfare,* 3-13.

Rotter, J.B. (1954). *Social learning and clinical psychology.* Englewood Cliffs, N.J.: Prentice Hall.

Rotter, J.B., Chance, J.E., & Phares, E.J. (1972). *Applications of a social learning theory of personality.* New York: Holt, Reinhart and Winston.

Stewart, R. (1977). Patients' attitudes to induction and labour. *British Medical Journal, 2,* 749-752.

Stokols, D. (1975). The reduction of cardiovascular risk: An application of social learning perspectives. *Behavioral Research Data Review Conference, Seattle, Washington, 1974,* American Heart Association.

Tanzer, D. (1972). *Why natural childbirth?* Garden City, New York: Doubleday.

Trethowan, W.H. & Conlon, M.F. (1965). The couvade syndrome. *American Journal of Psychiatry, 111,* 57-66.

Wallston, K.A., Kaplan, G.D., & Maides, S.A. (1976). Development and validation of the health locus of control (HLC) scale. *Journal of Consulting and Clinical Psychology, 44,* 4, 580-585.

Wallston, K.A., Maides, S.A., & Wallston, B.S. (1976). Health Related information seeking as a function of health-related locus of control and health value. *Journal of Research in Personality, 10,* 215-222.

Wallston, K.A. & Wallston, B.S. (1978). Development of the multi-dimensional health locus of control (MHLC) series. *Health Education Monographs, 6,* 2, 160-169.

Wheeler, A.S. (1977, October). Conduction anesthesia in obstetrics. *Journal of the American Association of Nurse Anesthetists, 45,* 494-499.

Selected Bibliography

Arms, S. (1975). *Immaculate deception.* Boston: Houghton Mifflin Co.

Bandura, A. (1971). *Social learning theory.* Morristown, N.J.: General Learning Press.

Chiota, B.J., Goolkasian, P., & Ladewig, P. (1976, January/February). Effects of separation from spouse in pregnancy, labor and delivery, and the postpartum period. *Journal of Obstetric-Gynecologic Nursing,* pp. 21-23.

Cobb, S. (1976). Social support as a moderation of life stress. *Psychosomatic Medicine, 38*(5), 300-312.

Crandon, A.J. (1978). Maternal anxiety and obstetric complications. *Journal of Psychosomatic Research, 23,* 109-111.

Davids, A., Devault, S., & Talmadge, M. (1961). Anxiety, pregnancy and childbirth abnormalities. *Journal of Consulting Psychology, 25,* 74-77.

Dick-Read, G. (1944). *Childbirth without fear.* New York: Harper and Row.

Edwards, A.L. (1957). *Techniques of attitude scale construction.* New York: Appleton-Century-Crafts.

Erickson, M.T. (1976a). The influence of health factors on psychological variables predicting complications of pregnancy, labor and delivery. *Journal of Psychosomatic Research, 20,* 21-24.

Erickson, M.T. (1965). Relationships between psychological attitudes during pregnancy and complications of pregnancy, labor and delivery (Summary). *Proceedings of the 73rd Annual Convention of the American Psychological Association, 1,* 213-214.

Erickson, M.T. (1966). The relationship between psychological variables and specific complications of pregnancy, labor and delivery. *Journal of Psychosomatic Research, 20,* 207-210.

Fawcett, J. (1978, July/August). Body image and the pregnant couple. *Maternal Child Nursing,* pp. 227-232.

Foster, Joyce Cameron (1981). Utah test for the childbearing year: Beliefs and perceptions about childbearing. Dissertation. University of Utah.

Green, L.W., Kreuter, M.W., Deeds, S.G., & Partridge, K.B. (1980). *Health education planning: A diagnostic approach.* Palo Alto, California: Mayfield Publishing Co.

Haire, D. (1972). *The cultural warping of childbirth.* Hillside, N.J.: International Childbirth Education Association.

Heinstein, M. (1967). Expressed attitudes and feelings of pregnant women and their relation to physical complications of pregnancy. *Merril-Palmer Quarterly, 1,* 217-236.

Henneborn, W.J., & Cogan, R. (1975). The effect of husband participation on reported pain and probability of medication during labor and birth. *Journal of Psychosomatic Research, 19,* 215-222.

Hollender, M.H., & McGehee, J.B. (1974). The wish to be held during pregnancy. *Journal of Psychosomatic Research, 18,* 193-197.

Howell, M.C. (1975). *Helping ourselves: Families and the human networks.* Boston: Beacon Press.

Kitzinger, S. (1962). *The experience of childbirth.* New York: Taplinger Publishing Co., Inc.

Lamaze, F. (1970). *Painless childbirth.* Chicago: Henry Regnery Co.

Lederman, R.P., Lederman, E., Work, B.A., & McCann, D.S. (1978). The relationship of maternal anxiety, plasma catacholamines and plasma cortisol to progress in labor. *American Journal of Obstetrics and Gynecology, 132*(5), 495-499.

Light, H.K., & Fenster, C. (1974). Maternal concerns during pregnancy. *American Journal of Obstetrics and Gynecology, 118*(1), 46-50.

Maiman, L.A., Becker, M.H., Kirscht, J.P., Haefner, D.P., & Drachman, R.H. (1977). Scales for measuring health belief model dimensions: A test of predictive value, internal consistency, and relationships among beliefs. *Health Education Monographs, 5*(3), 215-230.

Mason, J., & Brockert, J.E. (1980, November). *Utah Vital Statistics Annual Report, 1978.* Office of Health Planning and Policy Development, Utah State Department of Health.

McDonald, R.L. (1968). The role of emotional factors in obstetrics complications: A review. *Psychosomatic Medicine, 30*(2), 222-234.

Morris, N. (1968). Attitude survey in pregnancy. *Journal of Psychosomatic Research, 12,* 83-84.

Myers, R.E. (1977). Production of fetal asphyxia by maternal psychological stress. *Pavlovian Journal of Biological Science, 12*(1), 51-61.

Newton, R.W., Webster, P.A.C., Binu, P.A., Maskrey, N., & Phillips, A.B. (1979). Psychosocial stress in pregnancy and its relation to the onset of premature labor. *British Medical Journal, 2,* 411-413.

Nie, N.H., Hull, C.H., Jenkins, J.G., Steinbrenner, K., & Bent, D.H. (1975). *Statistical package for the social sciences* (2nd ed.). New York: McGraw-Hill.

Norr, K.L., Block, C.R., Charles, A., Myering, S., & Meyers, E. (1977). Explaining pain and enjoyment in childbirth. *Journal of Health and Social Behavior, 18,* 260-275.

Nunnally, J.C. (1978). Expectant fathers' perception of fathering. *American Journal of Nursing, 76*(9), 1440-1442.

Parlee, M.M. (1976). Social factors in the psychology of menstruation, birth and menopause. *Primary Care, 3*(3), 477-488.

Paten, H. (1966). The problem of routine circumcision. *Canadian Medical Association Journal, 95,* 576-581.

Peterson, G.H., Mehl, L.E., & Leiderman, H.P. (1979). The role of some birth-related variables in father attachment. *American Journal of Orthopsychiatry, 49*(2), 330-338.

Pies, H.E. (1976). The right of a father to be present in the delivery room. *American Journal of Public Health, 66*(7), 688-689.

Reid, K.E. (1975, Spring). Fatherhood and emotional stress: The couvade syndrome. *Journal of Social Welfare,* pp. 3-13.

Results are in: Utah health fair visitors mostly healthy. (1981, February). *Deseret News,* p. 2B.

Rotter, J.B. (1966). Generalized expectancies for internal versus external control of reinforcement. *Psychological Monographs, 80* (1, Whole No. 609).

Rotter, J.B. (1954). *Social learning and clinical psychology.* Englewood Cliffs, N.J.: Prentice Hall.

Rotter, J.B. (1975). Some problems and misconceptions related to the construct of internal versus external control of reinforcement. *Journal of Consulting and Clinical Psychology, 43*(1), 56-67.

Rotter, J.B., Chance, J.E., & Phares, E.J. (1972). *Applications of a social learning theory of personality.* New York: Holt, Reinhart and Winston.

Schaefer, E.S., & Manheimer, H. (1960, April). Dimensions of perinatal adjustment. *Eastern Psychological Association Meeting,* New York.

Shaw, R.A., & Robertson, W.O. (1963). Routine Circumcision: A problem for medicine. *American Journal of Diseases of Children, 106,* 216-217.

Stewart, R. (1977). Patients' attitudes to induction and labour. *British Medical Journal, 2,* 749-752.

Stokols, D. (1975). The reduction of cardiovascular risk: An application of social learning perspectives. *Behavioral Research Data Review Conference, Seattle Washington, 1974,* American Heart Association, 1975.

Tanzer, D. (1972). *Why natural childbirth?* Garden City, New York: Doubleday.

Throop, W.F., & McDonald, A.P. (1971). Internal-external locus of control: A bi liography. *Psychological Reports, 28,* 175-190.

Thurstone, L.L. (1929). Theory of attitude measurement. *Psychological Review, 36,* 222-241.

Trethowan, W.H., & Conlon, M.F. (1965). The couvade syndrome. *American Journal of Psychiatry, 111,* 57-66.

Wallston, K.A., Kaplan, G.D., & Maides, S.A. (1976). Development and validation of the health locus of control (HLC) scale. *Journal of Consulting and Clinical Psychology, 44*(4), 580-585.

Wallston, K.A., Maides, S.A., & Wallston, B.S. (1976). Health-related information seeking as a function of health-related locus of control and health value. *Journal of Research in Personality, 10,* 215-222.

Wallston, K.A., & Wallston, B.S. (1978). Development of the multi-dimensional health locus of control (MHLC) scales. *Health Education Monographs, 6*(2), 160-169.

Webster's Third New International Dictionary of the English Language, Unabridged. (1963). Boston: G & C Menian Co.

Westbrook, M.T. (1979). Socioeconomic differences in coping with childbearing. *American Journal of Community Psychology, 7*(4), 397-412.

Wheeler, A.S. (1977, October). Conduction anesthesia in obstetrics. *Journal of the American Association of Nurse Anesthetists. Vol. No. pp. 494-499.*

5
SUMMARY

Our research program proceeded for approximately six years funded by three different agencies and work completed in partial fulfillment of a PhD. We studied approximately 3500 women in the PIPAS Project and over 800 men and women in the Childbearing Year Project.

In the PIPAS project we developed and then revised to a short form a set of six stress scales (Social, Family, Financial, Work, Personal Habit Changes, and Lifestyle.) Concurrently we developed and revised to a short form a set of six symptom scales relative to the following systems (Gastrointestinal, Reproductive, Neuromuscular, Skin, and Cardiovascular Respiratory, plus a scale for General Adaptational Distress). We also developed an Illness Proneness Scale, which was later shortened to a Symptom Proneness scale. We used the 20 Psychiatric items of the Cornell Medical Index. We provided norms, reliabilities and intercorrelations for all these scales. Then we developed profile forms for the use of these scales for both pregnant women and their partners.

In PhD research one of us (JCH) developed the Utah Test for the Childbearing Year, which provided us with scales to measure Beliefs and Perceptions in five domains related to childbearing: Fear of the Childbirth Process, Childbirth Health Locus of Control, Personal Values About Childbearing and Childrearing, Passive Compliance versus Active Participation in Childbirth Care Decisions, and Father's Role and Responsibility in Childbearing. We obtained norms, reliabilities, and intercorrelations for these scales with primigravid women representative of the state of Utah.

A circumplex model was devised to place women in one of four categories: (a) High Childbearing Self-Competency and High Values About Childbearing and Childrearing, (b) High Childbearing Self-Competency and Low Values About Childbearing and Childrearing, (c) Low Childbearing Self-Competency and High Values About Childbearing and Childrearing, and (d) Low Childbearing Self-Competency and Low

Values About Childbearing and Childrearing. An individual profile form for the entire set of scales was also developed for use in the Childbearing Year Program.

Both sets of scales, PIPAS and Beliefs and Perceptions About Childbearing and Childrearing were used, and are being used in an educational program for expectant parents focused on development of high-level wellness during the period from conception through the first three months of parenting, i.e., the Childbearing Year. Longitudinal data were analyzed for this population of pregnant women.

Although there is some justification for the distinction between pure and applied research, we minimized the difference and are concerned primarily with clinically useful problem-solving. Our original idea was that:

1. Stress is primarily a motivational variable that intensifies above threshold common pregnancy symptoms or elicits sub-threshold symptoms.

2. Stress and symptom proneness both jointly not only intensify and energize symptoms, but interact so the effect of these variables is more than an additive sum.

3. Analysis of both sets of scales could provide a description of the pregnancy process in terms of the variables we would develop.

The hypotheses we draw from our work to date are many, but we shall discuss only two:

1. We would reclassify the customary division of pregnancy into trimesters into four time periods instead, each of which has its distinctive physiological and psychological tasks: (a) 0 to 3 months, (b) 4 to 6 months, (c) 7 and 8 months, (d) 9th month.

There is a quantitatve increase in the physiologic load throughout the nine months of pregnancy. During the fifth through the eighth month, the largest contributor to an increase in pregnancy symptoms are Symptom Proneness and CPI scores. This is a reflection of the woman's lifestyle prior to pregnancy, which continues into pregnancy at a slightly more intense level.

However, in the ninth month, there is a qualitative change. The major contributor to pregnancy symptoms is now the concurrent stresses as measured by the Stress Scales. It is clear from both path analyses and clinical data that the psychological and physiological problems of the ninth month are different from the seventh and eighth months.

We have developed a conception of the dynamics of the eighth and ninth month for the highly stressed women. Roughly, it is that an attitudinal/personality/cognitive integration is the first line of defense against stress. So long as there are attitudinal/personality/cognitive coping with stress possibilities, the physiological effects of stress are minimal. But for those pregnant women who are already physiologically stressed, the stresses by the eighth month strain the coping adaptation and deplete and exhaust the capability to adapt and integrate. In the ninth month, then, for these women stress results in increased pregnancy symptoms. These symptoms are signs that the integrative coping mechanisms are no longer working.

2. Result of our work has led us to conceptualize a phenomenon of pregnancy, which we call Adaptive Reserve. This reserve is influenced by both the physiological and the psychological state of the woman. The course of pregnancy represents a physiologic challenge to the woman as well as a psychological challenge. There is no doubt in our minds that most of these challenges are interrelated. If a woman has a large Adaptive Reserve she can cope with additional stresses. However, if a woman's Adaptive Reserve is low, then the addition of the increasing physiologic load of the fetus and pregnancy markedly affects the number and intensity of physical symptoms, and may lead to physical exhaustion and/or illness. Her Adaptive Reserve may be reduced by one or more of the following stressors: physical weakness or frailty; a crisis lifestyle with many psychological and outside stresses, poor personal management, and deficient coping skills; and beliefs and perceptions that affect her positive response to her health needs or add to her distress.

Therefore, if the Adaptive Reserve is low, the further burden of the physical demands of the pregnancy process may result in stress symptoms being highly manifest. In the stress-vulnerable woman, this may lead to illness; in the stress-resistant woman, it may reduce the quality of the pregnancy experience. Our therapeutic aim is to increase the Adaptive Reserve by controlling those variables that contribute to its depletion.

We aim to do this through a process which we call Stress Buffering. Stress Buffering involves high-level wellness enhancement by identification and management of *psychological* stresses through increased cognitive control, specific stress reduction activities, strengthening of personal support systems, establishment of an orderly routine of daily activities, and strategies to increase temporal resources (often available through community resources). Further Stress Buffering involves identification and management of *physiological* stresses through protective, toning, and aerobic exercise; nutrition; strategies for management of physical discomforts; and reduction of personal habits hazards and environmental hazards.

Because pregnancy is a process whose variables and their relations are constantly changing throughout the cycle, as evidenced by our path analyses, attention to these variables should be continuous throughout the childbearing experience. In addition, particular attention should be paid to the specific needs of women for additional psychological support during the second trimester, and for an increase of care of the highly stressed woman during the 9th month of pregnancy. Our expectation, based on our data, is that both the health of the woman and her fetus, as well as the quality of the pregnancy experience will be enhanced by Stress Buffering.

Our current model of Adaptive Reserve and Stress Buffering will influence our next steps of data acquisition and testing. We hope to gather data on these additional variables and subject them to regression and path analyses to identify further their respective weights in given circumstances.

Our test construction has served the dual purpose of (a) testing hypotheses and theories, and (b) developing practical instruments for clinical use. Although most clinical judgments are qualitative (i.e., x is an important factor), our measurement systems have allowed us to specify how important the clinical variables are. For example, clinically it can be observed that some babies are more healthy and active than others at birth. The APGAR score quantifies these observations. Similarly, mothers' responses to childbirth differ. What we need now is a "Mother APGAR."

Although we have the copyright on our scales, we offer them to anyone who wishes to use them in research or practice without further permission as long as they are credited to us. We would be most interested in the results of such use. The scales are to be used by the clinician not blindly, but as an aid in assessing pregnant women. If a pregnant woman reports many pregnancy symptoms in the absence of any delectable pathophysiology, the use of these instruments may indicate more precisely than general clinical judgment significant stress, symptom proneness, and psychological upset.

Bibliography

Abramson, J.H., Singh, A.R., & Mbambo, V. (1961). Antenatal stress and the baby's development. *Archives of Disease in Childhood, 36,* 42-49.

Aubry, R.H. & Nesbitt, R.E.L. (1969). High-risk obstetrics. *American Journal of Obstetrics and Gynecology, 105,* 2, 241-247.

Babson, S.G. & Denson, R.C. (1971). *Management of high-risk pregnancy and intensive care of the neonate.* St. Louis: Mosby.

Bandura, A. (1971). *Social learning theory.* Morristown, N.J.: General Learning Press.

Beck, J.C. & Worthen, K. (1972). Precipitating stress, crisis theory, and hospitalization in schizophrenia and depression. *Archives of General Psychiatry, 26,* 123-129.

Blau, A., Slaff, B., Easton, K., Welkowitz, J., Springarn, J., & Cohen, J. (1963). The psychogenic etiology of premature births. *Psychosomatic Medicine, 25,* 3, 201-211.

Burstein, I., Kinch, R.A.H., & Stern, L. (1974). Anxiety, pregnancy, labor and the neonate. *American Journal of Obstetrics and Gynecology, 118,* 2, 195-199.

Butler, N.R. (1963). *Perinatal mortality: The first report of the 1958 British perinatal mortality survey.* Edinburgh: E. & S. Livingstone, Ltd.

Butler, N.R. & Alberman, E.D. (Eds.) (1969). *Perinatal problems: The second report of the 1958 British perinatal mortality survey. Edinburgh: E. & S. Livingstone, Ltd.*

Cameron, J. (1979). Year-long classes for couples becoming parents. American Journal of Nursing, 6, 4, 358-362.

CLine, D.W. & Chosy, J.J. (1972). A prospective study of life changes and subsequent health changes. *Archives of General Psychiatry, 27,* 51-53.

Cobb, S. (1976). Social support as a moderation of life stress. *Psychosomatic Medicine, 38,* 5, 300-312.

Coddington, R.D. (1971). The significance of life events as etiological factors in the diseases of children. *Journal of Psychosomatic Research, 16,* 7-18.

Coddington, R.D. (1972). The significance of life events as etiological factors in the diseases of children — II. A study of a normal population. *Journal of Psychosomatic Research, 16,* 205-213.

Coddington, R.D. (1979). Life events associated with adolescent pregnancies. *Journal of Clinical Psychiatry, 40,* 180-185.

Cohen, J. (1969). *Statistical power analysis for the behavioral sciences.* New York: Academic Press.

Cooper, M. & Cooper, K.H. (1972). *Aerobics for women.* New York: Bantam Books (M. Evans & Co. Inc.).

Coppen, A.J. (1958). Psychosomatic aspects of pre-eclampic toxemia. *Journal of Psychosomatic Research, 2,* 241-265.

Davids, A. & DeVault, S. (1962). Maternal anxiety during pregnancy and childbirth abnormalities. *Psychosomatic Medicine, 24,* 5, 464-470.

Davids. A. & Rosengren, W.R. (1962). Social stability and psychological adjustment during pregnancy. *Psychosomatic Medicine, 24,* 6, 579-583.

Dohrenwend, B.S. (1973). Life events as stressors: A methodological inquiry. *Journal of Health & Social Behavior, 14,* 2, 167-175.

Downs, F. (1964). Maternal stress in primigravidas as a factor in the production of neonatal pathology. *Nursing Science, 2,* 348-367.

Edwards, A.L. (1957). *Techniques of attitude scale construction.* New York: Appleton-Century-Crofts.

Fagley, N., Miller, P., & Sullivan, J. (1982). Stress, symptom proneness, and general adaptational distress during pregnancy. *Journal of Human Stress, 6,* 15-22.

Friederich, M.A., Romano, J., & Lund, C.J. (1963). Psychologic aspects of obstetric-gynecologic practice. *American Journal of Obstetrics and Gynecology,* 1029-1033.

Gorsuch, R.L. & Key, M.K. (1974). Abnormalities of pregnancy as a function of anxiety and life stress. *Psychosomatic Medicine, 36,* 4, 352-362.

Green, L.W., Kreuter, M.W., Deeds, S.G., & Partridge, K.B. (1980). *Health education planning: A diagnostic approach.* Palo Alto, California: Mayfield Publishing Company.

Grimm, E.R. (1961). Psychological tension in pregnancy. *Psychosomatic Medicine, 23,* 6, 520-527.

Gunter, L.M. (1963). Psychopathology and stress in the life experience of mothers of premature infants. *American Journal of Obstetrics and Gynecology, 86,* 3, 333-340.

Hawkins, N.G., Davis, R., & Holmes, T.H. (1957). Evidence of psychosocial factors in the development of pulmonary tuberculosis. *American Review of Tuberculosis and Pulmonary Diseases, 75,* 5.

Heinstein, M. (1967). Expressed attitudes and feelings of pregnanty women and their relation to physical complications of pregnancy. *Merril-Palmer Quarterly, 1,* 217-236.

Helper, M.M., Cohen, R.L., Beiteman, E.T., & Eaton, L.F. (1968). Life-events and acceptance of pregnancy. *Journal of Psychosomatic Research, 12,* 183-188.

Hetzel, B.S., Bruer, B., & Poidevin, L.O.S. (1961). A survey of the relation between certain common antenatal complications in primiparae and stressful life situations during pregnancy. *Journal of Psychosomatic Research, 5,* 175-182.

Jacobson, E. (1964). *Anxiety and tension control.* Philadelphia: Lippincott.

Jones, A.C. (1978). Life changes and psychological distress as predictors of pregnancy outcome. *Psychosomatic Medicine, 40,* 5, 402-412.

Knoblock, H. & Pasamanick, B. (1960). Environmental factors affecting human development before and after birth. *Pediatrics,* 210-218.

Komaroff, A.L., Masuda, M., & Holmes, T.H. (1968). The social readjustment rating scale: A comparative study of Negro, Mexican, and White Americans. *Journal of Psychosomatic Research, 12,* 121.

Korones, S.B. (1972). *High Risk newborn infants: The basis for intensive nursing care.* St. Louis: Mosby.

Kuhn, T.S. (1962). *The structure of scientific revolutions.* Chicago: University of Chicago Press.

Lamaze, F. (1984). *Painless childbirth: The lamaze method.* Chicago: Contemporary Books, Inc.

Lewis, R., Charles, M., & Patwary, K.M. (1973). Relationships between birth weight and selected social, environmental, and medical care factors. *American Journal of Health, 63,* 11, 973-981.

Light, H.K., & Fenster, C. (1974). Maternal concerns during pregnancy. *Obstetrics and Gynecology, 132,* 5, 495-499.

Maiman, L.A., Becker, M.H., Kirscht, J.P., Haefner, D.P., & Drachman, R.H. (1977). Scales for measuring health belief model dimensions: A test of predictive value, internal consistency, and relationships among beliefs.

Health Education Monographs, 5, 3, 215-230.

Mason, J. & Brockert, J.E. (1980, November). *Utah Vital Statistics Annual Report, 1978.* Office of Health Planning and Policy Development, Utah State Department of Health.

Masuda, A.Z. & Holmes. T.H. (1967). The social readjustment rating scale: A cross-cultural study of Japanese and Americans. *Journal of Psychosomatic Research, 11,* 227.

McDonald, R.L. (1968). The role of emotional factors in obstetric complications: A review. *Psychosomatic Medicine, 30,* 222-237.

McDonald, R.L., Gynther, M.D., & Christakos, A.C. (1963). Relations between maternal anxiety and obstetric complications. *Psychosomatic Medicine, 25,* 4, 357-363.

Morris, N. (1968). Attitude survey in pregnancy. *Journal of Psychosomatic Research, 12,* 83-84.

Myers, J.K., Lindenthal, J.J., Pepper, M.P., & Ostrander, D.R. (1972). Life events and mental status: A longitudinal study. *Journal of Health and Social Behavior, 13,* 398-406.

Myrianthopoulas, N.C. & French, K.S. (1968). An application of the U.S. bureau of the census socioeconomic index to a large, diversified patient population. *Social Science & Medicine, 2,* 283-299.

Nam, C.B. & Powers, M.G. (1965). Variations in socioeconomic structure by race, residence and the life cycle. *American Sociological Review, 30,* 97.

Nie, H.H., Hull, C.H., Jenkins, J.G., Steinbrenner, K., & Bent, D.H. (1975). *Statistical package for the social sciences* (2nd ed.). New York: McGraw-Hill.

Niswander, K.R. & Gordon, M. (Eds.) (1972). *The women and their pregnancies.* Collaborative Perinatal Study of the National Institute of Neurological Disease and Stroke. Philadelphia: Saunders.

Norr, K.L., Block, C.R., Charles, A., Myering, S., & Meyers, E. (1977). Explaining pain and enjoyment in childbirth. *Journal of Health and Social Behavior, 18,* 260-275.

Nuckolls, K.B., Cassel, J., & Kaplan, B.H. (1972). Psychosocial assets, life crisis and the prognosis of pregnancy. *American Journal of Epidemiology, 95,* 5, 431-441.

Obrzut, L.A. (1976). Expectant fathers' perceptions of fathering. *American*

Journal of Nursing, 76, 9, 1440-1442.

Patten, H. (1966). The problem of routine circumcision. *Canadian Medical Association Journal, 95,* 576-581.

Paykel, E.S., Prusoff, B.A., Uhlenhuth, E.H. (1971). Scaling of life events. *Archives of General Psychiatry, 25,* 340-347.

Rahe, R.H. Meyer, M., Smith, M., Kjaer, G., & Holmes, T.H. (1964). Social stress and illness onset. *Journal of Psychosomatic Research, 8,* 35-44.

Results are in: Utah health fair visitors mostly healthy (1981, February). *Deseret News,* 2B.

Roghmann, K.J. & Haggerty, R.J. (1973). Daily stress, illness, and use of health services in young families. *Pediatric Research, 7,* 520-526.

Rotter, J.B. (1966). Generalized expectancies for internal versus external control of reinforcement. *Psychological Monographs, 80,* (1, Whole No. 609).

Rotter, J.B. (1975). Some problems and misconceptions related to the construct of internal versus external control of reinforcement. *Journal of Consulting and Clinical Psychology, 43,* 1, 56-57.

Satin, D.C. (1972). (Help): Life stresses and psycho-social problems in the hospital emergency unit. *Social Psychiatry, 7,* 119-126.

Schaefer, E.S., & Manheimer, H. (1960, April). Dimensions of perinatal adjustment. *Eastern Psychological Association Meeting,* New York.

Schwartz, J.L. (1973). A study of the relationship between maternal life change events and premature delivery. Unpublished Master's Thesis. University of Washington.

Shaw, R.A., & Robertson, W.O. (1963). Routine circumcision: A problem for medicine. *American Journal of Diseases of Children, 106,* 216-217.

Smith, A.C., Flick, G.L., Ferriss, G.S., & Sellmann, A.H. (1972). Prediction of developmental outcome at seven years from prenatal, perinatal, and postnatal events. *Child Development, 43,* 495-507.

Smith, W.G. (1971). Critical life-events and prevention strategies in mental health. *Archives of General Psychiatry, 25,* 102-109.

Stott, D.H. (1958). Some psychosomatic aspects of casualty in reproduction. *Journal of Psychosomatic Research, 3,* 42-55.

Stott, D.H. (1974). Follow-up study from birth on the effects of prenatal stress. *Developmental Medicine and Child Neurology, 118,* 2, 195-199.

Thomson, K.C. & Medrie, H.C. (1972). Environmental stress in primary depressive illness. *Archives of General Psychiatry, 26,* 130-132.

Throop, W.F., & McDonald, A.P. (1971). Internal-external locus of control: A bibliography. *Psychological Reports, 28,* 175-190.

Thurlow, H.J. (1971). Illness in relation to life situation and sick role tendency. *Journal of Psychosomatic Research, 15,* 73.

Thurstone, L.L. (1929). Theory of attitude measurement. *Psychological Review, 36,* 222-241.

Uhlenhuth, E.H. & Paykel, E.S. (1973). Symptom intensity and life events. *Archives of General Psychiatry, 28,* 473-477.

Webster's Third New International Dictionary of the English Language, Unabridged (1963). Boston: G & C Menian Company.

Westbrook, M.T. (1979). Socioeconomic differences in coping with childbearing. *American Journal of Community Psychology, 7,* 4, 397-412.

APPENDIX A

The Pregnancy Illness Proneness and Stress Scales (PIPAS): The Childbearing Year Assessment Packet for Pregnant Women

PLEASE READ AND SIGN THIS CONSENT FORM BEFORE COMPLETING THE PERSONAL HEALTH PROFILE PACKET. THANK YOU.

ID#________

Childbearing Year Program

University of Utah College of Nursing

Information

Purpose:

Your personal health profile is designed to:

1. Give you information which may assist you in health care decisions,
2. Help your group leader to individualize the childbearing year classes to your groups' needs and interests,
3. Provide information to enable health professionals to plan programs to meet the health needs of expectant and new parents.

The profile consists of four parts:

1. Nutritional Status
2. Physical Fitness Status
3. General Health Status
4. Utah Test Appraising Health — Stress Status

Filling out the above forms will enable us to prepare for you a computerized nutrition printout, a lifestress profile, and information concerning your health and fitness status. Please ask any questions you wish for further clarification from the person supplying this form.

All information will be kept confidential and you will not be identified in any way in subsequent research summaries of the data.

Consent

I have read the foregoing and my questions have been answered. I desire to participate in this study and give permission to the scientists at the College of Nursing to analyze and summarize the data and provide me with the information listed above.

________________________ ________________________

Date Signature

This program is/has been supported by P.H.S. Grant MC-R-490355-02, March of Dimes Grants CHE-34/11-32 and CHE-33/11-54, and Department of HEW Division of Nursing Grant NU 28028-01. The contents of this survey are not the responsibility of the awarding parties.

ID#______

Utah Test Appraising Health — IVS

Pregnancy, Illness Proneness, and Stress (PIPAS Profile)

INSTRUCTIONS: Please circle the illnesses or symptoms you have had within the past ten years.

Example:

1. Gas
(2.) Stomach cramps
3. Gallbladder trouble
(4.) Hemorrhoids (piles)
(5.) Crampy pain in abdomen
6. Trouble with teeth/gums

This means you have had stomach cramps, hemorrhoids (piles), and a crampy pain in your abdomen within the past ten years, but have not had gas, gallbladder trouble or trouble with teeth/gums.

Remember: If the term is not applicable, you make no mark on the sheet.

Please circled the illnesses or symptoms you have had within the past ten years.

1. Gas
2. Stomach cramps
3. Gallbladder trouble
4. Hemorrhoids (piles)
5. Crampy pain in abdomen
6. Trouble with teeth/gums
7. Loss of appetite for more than a day
8. Burning sensation in stomach
9. Sensitive to particular foods
10. Earaches
11. Trouble with eyes
12. Prolonged stuffy nose
13. Severe headaches
14. Hay fever
15. Tonsillitis
16. Persistent cold in chest
17. Urinary tract infections
18. Bladder infections
19. Blood in urine
20. High or low blood pressure
21. Anemia
22. Bleeding tendency
23. Allergies
24. Chest pains
25. Persistent cough
26. Feeling of general weakness
27. Gain or loss of weight (more than 10#)
28. Severe menstrual cramps
29. Stiff or sore joints
30. Specific muscle weakness
31. Cuts or wounds which healed slowly
32. Bruise easily

INSTRUCTIONS: Please circle the period(s) during THIS pregnancy in which you OFTEN have had or are having any of the following symptoms.

If you are 3 months pregnant circle applicable items in the first column only.

If you are 4 to 6 months pregnant circle applicable items in both the first and second columns.

If you are 7 months pregnant circle applicable items in all three columns.

Example:

	When 1-3 Months Pregnant	When 4-6 Months Pregnant	When 7-9 Months Pregnant
33. Loss of appetite for some time	(A)	A	(A)
34. Frequent dry mouth-bad breath	A	A	A
35. Frequent constipation	A	(A)	A

This means you OFTEN had loss of appetite for some time when 1-3 Months Pregnant and 7-9 Months Pregnant but not when 4-6 Months Pregnant; you did not experience frequent dry mouth-bad breath during any of your pregnancy; and you had frequent constipation when 4-6 Months Pregnant but not when 1-3 Months Pregnant or 7-9 Months Pregnant.

Remember: 1. If the item is not applicable, you make no mark on the sheet, and
2. You may mark more than one response for each symptom.

	When 1-3 Months Pregnant	When 4-6 Months Pregnant	When 7-9 Months Pregnant
33. Loss of appetite for some time	A	A	A
34. Frequent dry mouth-bad breath	A	A	A
35. Frequent constipation	A	A	A
36. Certain foods bother you	A	A	A
37. Troubled by nausea or morning sickness	A	A	A
38. Troubled with vomiting (other than No. 37)	A	A	A
39. Heartburn	A	A	A
40. Stomach cramps	A	A	A
41. Crave certain foods	A	A	A
42. Frequent frightening dreams	B	B	B
43. Felt persistently tired	B	B	B
44. Not much energy	B	B	B
45. Increase in nervous irritability	B	B	B

	When 1-3 Months Pregnant	When 4-6 Months Pregnant	When 7-9 Months Pregnant
46. More sensitive to light, sounds, smell	B	B	B
47. Trouble getting to sleep	B	B	B
48. Trouble staying asleep	B	B	B
49. Felt persistently tired	B	B	B
50. Headaches	B	B	B
51. Persistent increase in vaginal discharge without itching or burning	C	C	C
52. Painful breasts	C	C	C
53. Tingling in breasts	C	C	C
54. Increased breast size	C	C	C
55. Contraction of uterus, sometimes associated with discomfot, pain	C	C	C
56. Sharp pains in lower abdomen on either side when you suddenly change positions	C	C	C
57. Do you feel stretched out of shape?	C	C	C
58. Need to pass urine (water) frequently	C	C	C
59. Pain or burning feeling during/following urination (passing water)	C	C	C
60. Muscle cramps especially at night	D	D	D
61. Low backache	D	D	D
62. Stiff or sore joints	D	D	D
63. Aching in arms/legs	D	D	D
64. Numbness in arms/legs	D	D	D
65. Weakness in arms/legs	D	D	D
66. Have a tendency to drop things	D	D	D
67. Pains in rib cage	D	D	D
68. Have difficulty walking	D	D	E
69. Hands often sweaty	E	E	E
70. Definite rashes	E	E	E
71. Itchy skin	E	E	E
72. Perspire a great deal	E	E	E
73. Skin blotches	E	E	E
74. Marked changes in hair	E	E	E
75. Skin infections	E	E	E
76. Bruise easily	E	E	E

	When 1-3 Months Pregnant	When 4-6 Months Pregnant	When 7-9 Months Pregnant
77. Stretch marks on breasts, abdomen, hips	E	E	E
78. Frequently feel heart pounding	F	F	F
79. Frequently feel short of breath	F	F	F
80. Need to sleep on two or more pillows	F	F	F
81. Get "colds" frequently	F	F	F
82. Troubled by stuffy nose	F	F	F
83. Frequent cough day or night	F	F	F
84. Swelling in ankles and legs	F	F	F
85. Swelling of hands/face late in the day	F	F	F
86. Frequently feel hot and flushed	F	F	F
87. Did/do you get nervous and shaky when approached by someone you consider to be important?	G	G	G
88. Did/do you usually feel unhappy and depressed?	G	G	G
89. Did/does life look entirely hopeless?	G	G	G
90. Did/do you suffer from severe nervous exhaustion?	G	G	G
91. Did/does every little thing get on your nerves lately and wear you out?	G	G	G
92. Did/do you often become suddenly scared for no good reason?	G	G	G
93. Did/do you often wish you were dead and away from it all?	G	G	G
94. Did/does your thinking get completely mixed up when you have to do things quickly?	G	G	G
95. Were/are you constantly keyed up and jittery?	G	G	G
96. Did/do frightening thoughts keep coming back in your mind?	G	G	G
97. Did/do you often get spells of of complete exhaustion or fatigue?	G	G	G
98. Were/are you often bothered by thumping of the heart?	G	G	G
99. Did/do you wear yourself out worrying about your health?	G	G	G

	When 1-3 Months Pregnant	When 4-6 Months Pregnant	When 7-9 Months Pregnant
100. Did/does your heart often race like mad?	G	G	G
101. Did/does pressure or pain in the head often make life miserable for you?	G	G	G
102. Did/do you wish you always had someone at your side to advise you?	G	G	G
103. Did/do you go to pieces if you don't constantly control yourself?	G	G	G
104. Did/do you often shake or tremble?	G	G	G
105. Did/does worrying continually get you down?	G	G	G
106. Were/are you considered to be a nervous person?	G	G	G

INSTRUCTIONS: The following questions are to be answered by circling the appropriate column. If the item is not applicable, do not respond at all. If the item is applicable, please respond by circling the first column for six to twelve months ago and the second column for during the past six months.

Remember: 1. If the item is not applicable, you make no mark on the sheet, and
2. You may mark more than one response for each item.

Please respond to the following questions by circling the first or second or first and second columns if they apply to you during one or both of the two periods in the last year.

	Six To Twelve Months Ago	During The Past Six Months
107. Have you had a change in your role as wife or mother?	A	A
108. Have you had a change in living conditions?	B	B
109. Have you changed some of your personal habits?	C	C
110. Have you had a change in responsibilities at work?	D	D
111. Have you experienced a marital reconciliation?	A	A
112. Have you had a change in residence?	B	B
113. Have you changed some of your eating habits?	C	C
114. Have you had a fight with a close friend?	E	E
115. Do you have monthly car payments?	F	F
116. Have you begun or finished school?	B	B
117. Have you changed some of your sleeping habits?	C	C
118. Have you been either drunk or disorderly?	E	E
119. Have you had a change in attitude toward your job?	D	D
120. Have you gotten married?	A	A
121. Do you have a bank loan (other than education, house, or car loan)?	F	F
122. Have you had a change in your usual social activities?	B	B
123. Have you changed some of your execise habits?	C	C
124. Have you left home for a period of hours or longer because of a dispute?	E	E

	Six To Twelve Months Ago	During The Past Six Months
125. Have you had a change in your boss?	D	D
126. Have you had trouble with your in-laws?	A	A
127. Have you changed your recreational activities?	C	C
128. Have you had a change in your co-workers?	D	D
129. Have you had more or fewer arguments with your spouse?	A	A
130. Have you had a change in your physical conditions at work?	D	D
131. Have you had an increase in family income?	F	F
132. Have you run away from home?	E	E
133. Have you discussed a possible separation from your spouse?	A	A
134. Have you had a change in your financial state?	F	F
135. Have you changed the time you wake up or go to bed?	C	C
136. Have you had a close friend who has been arrested or jailed?	E	E
137. Have you had a temporary change in the kind of work you do?	D	D
138. Have you had religious conflicts within your household?	A	A
139. Have you recently made a major purchase (house, furniture, car, etc.)?	F	F
140. Have you had a change in the time (more or less) you spend by yourself?	B	B
141. Have you occasionally used social drugs (marijuana, alcohol)?	E	E
142. Because of inflation, have you changed your eating habits?	F	F
143. Have you thought of suicide?	E	E
144. If you have a checking account, have you overdrawn it?	F	F
145. Have you been spending less time in outdoor activities?	B	B
146. Have you increased or decreased social contacts?	C	C

	Six To Twelve Months Ago	During The Past Six Months
147. Have you experienced a change of attitude toward your family?	A	A
148. Have you watched television or read more than before your wife's pregnancy?	B	B
149. Have you changed your work hours or work conditions?	D	D
150. Have you changed from thinking of your wife as a pregnant woman to being the mother of an unborn baby?	B	B
151. Have you experienced considerable mood changes?	C	C
152. Have you become fearful of being alone while at home?	E	E
153. Have you strongly disliked your work?	D	D
154. Have you had arguments about family finances?	A	A
155. Have you bought major purchases on credit?	F	F
156. Has there been a change in your financial state?	F	F
157. Have you changed your style of dressing?	B	B
158. Have you exceeded the speed limit by more than 10 miles per hour?	E	E
159. Have you wanted to quit your present job (if you could afford not to work)?	D	D
160. Have you had a change in your daily activities?	C	C

1. Who is the chief earner of income in your family? (please check one)

   ______ Husband ______ Wife ______ Other ______ Equal

2. What is the yearly income for your family from all sources? (please check one)

______ None	______ $ 9,000-10,000	______ $19,000-20,999
______ $1,000-2,999	______ $11,000-12,999	______ $21,000-22,999
______ $3,000-4,999	______ $13,000-14,999	______ $23,000 or more
______ $5,000-6,999	______ $15,000-16,999	
______ $7,000-8,999	______ $17,000-18,999	

3. What is the highest level of education achieved by: (please check one for each)

	Female Head Household	Male Head Household
0-6 grades, ungraded	______	______
7-9 grades, Junior High School	______	______
10-11 grades, some High School	______	______
Graduate, High School	______	______
At least one year College	______	______
Graduate, four year College	______	______
Post graduate, College	______	______

4. What is the occupation of the female head of the household? (please check one)

______ Student in High School, Trade School	______ Salesman
______ Laborer, farm laborer	______ Clerical
______ Other service worker	______ Proprietor, manager, business or agriculture
______ Domestic worker	______ Professional, including college student
______ Operator	
______ Craftsman	

5. What is the occupaion of the male head of household? (please check one)

_______ Student in High School, Trade School
_______ Laborer, farm laborer
_______ Other service worker
_______ Domestic worker
_______ Operator
_______ Craftsman
_______ Salesman
_______ Clerical
_______ Proprietor, manager, business or agriculture
_______ Professional, including college students

6. Was this pregnancy planned? (please check one)

_______ Yes _______ No

7. Did you breast feed your last baby? (please check one)

_______ Yes _______ No

8. Do you plan to breast feed this baby? (please check one)

_______ Yes _______ No

9. Has this pregnancy so far been (a) easier than you expected, (b) what you expected, or (c) harder than you expected? (please check one)

ID #______

GENERAL HEALTH STATUS

1. What is your age? ______
2. What is your marital status? Single ______ Married ______ Widow ______ Divorced ______ Sep ______
3. Health history:
   Significant family history? No ______ Yes ______ If yes, explain ______
   ____
   Significant health problems (yourself)? No ______ Yes ______ If yes, explain
   ____
   Allergies (yourself)? No ______ Yes ______ If yes, please list ______
   ____
4. Personal habits history: (If *less* than once a day usage, fill in for week only.)

   Smoking? No ______ Cigarettes, pipes, cigars ______/day OR ______/week

   Alcohol? No ______ Number of ounces ______/day OR ______/week
   (1 mixed drink = 1 oz. alcohol
   1 beer [12 oz., Utah] = 1/3 oz. alcohol)

   Caffeine? No ______ cups coffee ______/day OR ______ cups/week

   No ______ cups cocoa ______/day OR ______ cups/week

   No ______ 12 oz. cola drinks ______/day OR ______/week
   (include Pepsi, Coke, Mountain Dew, Tab, etc.)

   No ______ chocolate bars (individual size) ______/day OR ______/week

   No ______ cups tea ______/day OR ______ cups/week

   Seat belt usage? Never ______ Occasionally ______ Most of time ______ Always ______

4. *(continued)*

Drugs and medications used in the last 6 months: (list name, dose, frequency)

Prescribed Drugs (ex. insulin, sleeping pills)	Non Prescription Drugs (ex. aspirin, vitamins)	Social Drugs (ex. barbiturates, marijuana)

5. Obstetric History: Baby due date ____________

Dates of Previous Pregnancy Terminations	Birthweights OR What Month of Pregnancy for Abortion/Miscarriage

Total Length of Labor (Hours)	Pregnancy, Labor, Delivery or Baby Complications (State *no* or explain)

ID # ________

PHYSICAL FITNESS PROFILE

Date ________

I Sports/Activities

How much time did you spend in the following activities?

0 = Virtually no time; 1 = Less than average; 2 = Greater than average; 3 = Great deal of time.

Activity	Childhood (6-12)	Adolescence (13-18)	Adult (19 +)
Badminton	________	________	________
Baseball	________	________	________
Bicycling	________	________	________
Bowling	________	________	________
Calesthenics	________	________	________
Cheerleading	________	________	________
Dance	________	________	________
Football	________	________	________
Gymnastics	________	________	________
Hiking	________	________	________
Hockey	________	________	________
Ice Skating	________	________	________
Roller Skating	________	________	________
Running	________	________	________
Skiing	________	________	________
Swimming	________	________	________
Tennis/Racket Sports	________	________	________
Track and Field	________	________	________
Volleyball	________	________	________
Yoga	________	________	________

II Current Aerobic Activities

Please check *current* endurance activities and record the approximate times per week spent doing each and usual total minutes each time.

Activity	Average Times Per Week	Usual Total Minutes Each Time
Walk Briskly	________	________
Jog	________	________
Run	________	________
Skip Rope	________	________
Swim	________	________
Bicycle	________	________
Tennis/Racket Sports	________	________
Skiing	________	________
Skating	________	________
Volleyball	________	________

III. Height _______ Current weight _______ Non pregnant weight _______

---------DO NOT WRITE BELOW THIS LINE---------

IV. Resting Pulse

1st Class ________ 8th Class ________ 10th Class ________

Date __________ Date __________ Date __________

UTAH-IVS CODING KEY

Question Number	Category	Columns Used
1 - 32	SP	A
33 - 41	GI	C 1st trimester D 2nd trimester E 3rd trimester
42 - 50	GAD	same
51 - 59	REPR	same
60 - 68	NM	same
69 - 77	SKIN	same
78 - 86	CVR	same
87 - 106	CPI	same
114, 118, 124, 132, 136, 141, 143, 152, 158	SOCSTR	D 6 - 12 months ago E 0 - 6 months ago
110, 119, 125, 128, 130, 138, 149, 153, 159	WRKSTR	same
107, 111, 120, 126, 129, 133, 138, 147, 154	FAMSTR	same
115, 121, 131, 134, 139, 142, 144, 155, 156	FINSTR	same
108, 112, 116, 122, 140, 145, 148, 150, 157	STYSTR	same
109, 113, 117, 123, 127, 135, 146, 151, 160	PERSTR	same

APPENDIX B

The Prediction of Second Trimester Pregnancy Symptoms

We have engaged in what we call locally a "stepwise research program." That is, we have developed sequentially in a stepwise fashion our measuring instruments and conceptual systems related to stress and pregnancy. When we had reached one step or level of conceptual formulation then we were able to develop new measures. New measures showed us new relationships, which allowed us to develop our conceptual notions and to start the cycle of development again, but at a higher level of precision. Occasionally we were led astray by our theoretical pre-conceptions and occasionally we went up some measurement blind alleys. Another image of our progress, more biologically oriented, is that the PIPAS Project represented an amoebic like organism; thrusting out pseudopodia; meeting obstacles some of which were dissolved and incorporated, others indigestible and put aside; making progress in a general direction. Whatever the imagery, our actual progress is best seen retrospectively in this general survey.

Dependent Variables

Our ultimate dependent variables are baby and mother outcomes of labor and delivery. The immediate precursors of these are the actual labor and delivery variables. And the precursors of these are symptoms during pregnancy. Our first approach was simply to survey pregnancy symptoms of women who took our survey forms. Rather quickly we separated the women and the symptoms into trimesters. We can also ask how does a woman in her second trimester report her second trimester symptoms? How does a woman in the third trimester report her second and her third trimester symptoms? The next stage of our development was to develop six categories into which these symptoms could be classified so that we could get seven indices, six of general systems — Gastrointestinal, Skin, Neuromuscular, Cardiovascular/Respiratory, Reproductive, and a category of our own construction, General Adaptational Distress — and an index that was simply the total number of symptoms reported for the trimester. The symptoms were classified into these categories with the help of Sally Yeomans, R.N., C.N.M., the PIPAS Project Midwife Consultant.

A factor analytic study of symptoms each trimester showed that there were three factors, one for each trimester, and that the best single symptom measure for each trimester is the total number of symptoms for that trimester. Before we had done this analysis we had speculated idly that the GI symptoms would probably be best for the first trimester, the cardiovascular/respiratory would come through strong in the third trimester. For our data, however, the total number of symptoms a woman has is the best index of each trimester factor. And of the total symptoms for each trimester, the best of these was the second trimester, which had the largest variance. Consequently, we have used this as our primary dependent variable in our preliminary studies.

We have also found that not all of the 53 symptoms of our pregnancy symptoms are stress sensitive. So we constructed a regression equation with our best stress index (Total) combined with the Symptom Proneness and the Cornell Psychiatric Index. This regression score was then correlated with each of the pregnancy symptoms.

Then we took the 15 items with the highest correlation with the regression score and computed a Kuder-Richardson Formula 20 reliability coefficient. Next we added 5 more items, then computed the reliability of the scale. Finally, we took the top 30 items in terms of regression score/symptom correlation and computered the KR-20. These reliabilities can be seen in Table 1. We selected as our criterion measure the 20-item scale and called it the "SIV220" (Stress Illness Vulnerability, second trimester, 20 items). The SIV220 items are presented in Table 2.

Independent Measures

The basic thrust of our early research reported here was (a) to find the relations of a general measure of stress, the *Schedule of Recent Experience* (SRE) scores to second trimester pregnancy symptoms, and then (b) do better. We have discussed the rationale of our approach in Chapter 1. The basic consideration was that the predictive performance of a general survey form can be improved considerably when the items on the survey are closely fitted to the population of interest. Thus we constructed stress scales that were based upon the responses of pregnant women, rather than on the broad population sample, which was the norm group for the SRE. We also broke the stresses down into six stress scales so that reliable estimates of different stresses could be obtained. These, in turn, could be combined optimally in regression equations.

Our baseline data is the study of 299 pregnant women who took the SRE while attending prenatal classes and were given a set of symptom items. The highest correlation was .37. It is to be noted, that subsequently we developed a set of 53 symptoms categorized into six classes. The symptom scale of the baseline study using the SRE is not the same symptom list as used in the following studies. The first symptom list, however, served as the basis for the subsequent revision so there is a considerable overlap between the two lists of symptoms. We are not making a strong argument about the differences between the first and second symptom lists correlations. Here we are concerned to show the progressive growth of the correlation coefficients as we increase the scope of our measurement system.

We report a series of statistical studies based upon 255 women who were in the second trimester and reported their second trimester symptoms. Their demographic characteristics can be seen in Table 3.

Stage 1

The correlations of the scores for the individual stress scale and the two dependent measures, the total number of symptoms for the second trimester and the SIV220 can be seen in Stage I of Table 4. Here it is apparent that the order of importance of the stresses in predicting symptoms is as follows:

Personal Habit Stress
Family Stress
Social Stress
Life Style Stress
Financial Stress
Work Stress

This finding is in general accord with clinical opinions on these matters. Of great interest statistically is that in Stage II, when these stresses are combined in a regression equation, then the multiple correlation (.4477) is not much higher than the correlation of Personal Habit Stress with the total symptoms. This means, in effect, that there is not much independent variance being added by those other scales to the Personal Habit Stress in the multiple correlations.

We have a theory that there is a casual chain of the following sort:

Secondary	Primary	Personal		
Group------->	Group--->	Stresses---->	Symptoms--->	Illnesses
Stresses	Stresses		(Physiological	
(Sociological)	(Family)	(Psychological)	Stress)	

This simple model would imply that casually adjacent factors would be more closely correlated than casually distant factors. Thus we expect our best predictions of variations in labor and delivery to be our SIV320 —our 20-item stress illness vulnerability scale for the third trimester. At the other end of the casual chain we also expect stress of a sociological sort to be more closely related to psychological stress indices than to physiological stresses.

We are now able to do some preliminary testing of these hypotheses. We look on the Financial, Work, and Social Stress scales as fundamentally sociological in character. These have, as noted above, the lower correlations with pregnancy symptoms than the other scales. When we did partial correlations between these stresses in which we partialled Family, Lifestyle, and Personal Habit Change Stresses out of the relations of Social, Work, and Financial Stresses to second trimester pregnancy symptoms the correlations dropped to around zero. There was a slight indication that work stress might still have a slight relation (P .082, one-tailed test of significance) to second trimester pregnancy symptoms. (See table 5.)

Stage II

Our general research approach is to use regression analyses. The basic rationale of constructing a number of stress scales in Stage I was not only to have reliable measures of particularly important stresses, but to be able to determine the differential weights of the stresses when combined in regression equations in either a planned theoretical or a stepwise order.

Our experience with the fluctuation of constants with these regressions as samples change, however, has led us from early optimism to a present profound skepticism about any regression weights based upon less than 200 cases. Our basic method is, as in the case of the intra-individual pattern of stresses resulting in illnesses that the clinician assesses, to look for inter-individual patterns of stresses that have characteristic symptom outcomes.

We interpret the partial correlation as indicating that social, work, and financial stresses, when the common variance shared with the other stresses is removed, has little relation to second trimester symptoms for this sample of subjects.

This conclusion is merely restating the statistical implications, but it is rather striking in its content. The health care literature has many references to the fact that people in the lower socioeconomic-educational level tend to have more illnesses, more severe illnesses, and recover more slowly from illnesses than their higher socioeconomic-educational cohorts. We have maintained as an ideological position that it is not the category of socioeconomic-education level that is so important. The stresses associated with these lower levels do the damage. We could think of persons in the lower levels not badly stressed, i.e., well adapted, who are relatively symptom free. On the other end, there are many highly stressed, symptom-prone individuals in the higher socioeconomic-education levels. The finding of this set of partial correlations is even more radical. It is that the stresses that are sociological in nature relate significantly to symptoms/illnesses, but probably due to the mediation of familial and personal stresses. When these primary group and psychological stresses are partialled out of the relations of the sociological stresses with symptoms, the correlations drop to approximately zero. Our simple conceptual model is looking better as we amass more relevant data.

Stage III

In Stage III we combined the regression score obtained from Stage II with the Symptom Proneness Index. Originally we were working with a theory of illness proneness, but, after we constructed our scale and used it for a time, it dawned on us that we were really checking symptoms and trying to predict prenatal symptoms in this phase of our study. For the contents of the Symptom Proneness Index see Chapter 1. The total number of symptoms reported is the Symptom Proneness Index. The mean and standard deviation of the scale for this study are: x = 6.471, SD = 3,907, N = 255.

Due to the jump in the multiple correlation from Stage II (.4477) to Stage III (.5672) we conclude that the Symptom Proneness Index is adding a lot of independent variance to the stress variance. That is to say that the multiple correlation increases substantially as variables which are correlated with the criterion (pregnancy symptoms) but which are relatively independent of stresses. The history of physical symptoms is different in kind from sociological and psychological stresses as we measure them.

Stage IV

In Stage IV we added to our previous regression equation the scores of the Cornell Psychiatric Index. This is a 20-item scale that is part of the Cornell Medical Inventory, which has been widely used in health research. The contents of this scale are in Chapter 1. There are four of these psychosomatic questions:

Did/do you often get spells of complete exhaustion or fatigue?

Were/are you often bothered by thumping of the heart?

Did/does your heart often race like mad?

Did/does pressure or pain in the head often make life miserable for you?

These items, of course, have a basic similarity with some of the symptoms a woman would report in the second trimester. This fact points in two directions: (a) the physiological states associated with psychological difficulty are energized in pregnancy so that the associated tension, panic, and depressed feeling states are probably easily elicited in the presence of this underlying physiological condition, and (b) if a person has these underlying physiological states but is pregnant, interpretation of them cannot be given as if she has them and is not pregnant. We believe both of these statements are probably true.

At any event, knowing the overlap of the psychosomatic items with our symptom scales we combined the CPI with our previous regression equation of Stage III and found that the multiple correlation had a substantial increase (to .7095, 50% of variance explained). As is well known, increases of this magnitude are hard to obtain particularly when the initial correlation is, as it was in Stage III .57 (the higher the correlation coefficient the harder it is to add increments). The mean and standard deviation of this sample was: x = 2.388, SD = 2.885, N = 255, KR-20 = .80.

When we computed the multiple correlation with the four psychosomatic items left out of the CPI measure, the KR-20 reliability of the scale was .7844. With this 16-item CPI scale the multiple correlation in Stage IV were General Illness Predisposition Index with Total 2nd Trimester Symptoms = .6846 and with Stress Sensitive Symptom Scale, Second Trimester = .7018 (N - 255 for both correlations). Thus we can be reasonably sure that the increment in the multiple correlation in Stage IV is not due to commonality of psychosomatic symptoms with pregnancy symptoms, but is due to the contribution of general psychological difficulties to the experience of severe second trimester pregnancy symptoms.

At one point we looked upon the CPI as measuring psychological stress, which was parallel to the physiological stress as measured by the number of stress related symptoms (SIV220). A symptom-prone, stressed person might have two manifestations of this condition: (a) psychological symptoms as measured by the CPI or (b) physiological symptoms as measured by our SIV220. With our present model, however, we look upon the psychological states both as casual factors in symptoms and as feedback phenomena from physiological symptoms.

TABLE 1.

The Correlations of the Stress Illness Vulnerability Scales (SIV) with the General Illness Predisposition Index (Stress Index plus Symptom Proneness Index plus the Cornell Psychiatric Item Index) N=255

	Multiple Correlation
General Illness Predisposition Index with SIV215	.7141
General Illness Predisposition Index with SIV220	.7328
General Illness Predisposition Index with SIV225	.7339
General Illness Predisposition Index with SIV230	.7202

SIV215 = Stress Illness Vulnerability, Second Trimester Symptoms, 15 Item Test
SIV220 = Stress Illness Vulnerability, Second Trimester Symptoms, 20 Item Test

NOTE: We selected SIV220 as our measure and ran correlations of our various indices with it as shown in Table 4. The particular items of SIV220 are given in Table 2.

TABLE 2.

SIV220 Items

In the Utah-IV test, the basic stem question and the items of the SIV220 are as follows:

Please indicate if while 4 to 6 months pregnant you OFTEN have had or are having any of the following symptoms.

1.	GI202	Frequent dry mouth - bad breath
2.	GI205	Certain foods bother you
3.	GI210	Gas
4.	GAD202	Ill health frequently affecting your work
5.	GAD207	Increase in nervous irritability
6.	GAD209	Trouble getting to sleep
7.	GAD210	Trouble staying asleep
8.	REPR207	Increased breast size
9.	REPR210	Sharp pains in lower abdomen on either side when you suddenly change position
10.	REPR212	Do you feel stretched out of shape?
11.	REPR213	Need to pass urine (water) frequently?
12.	NM203	Stiff or sore joints
13.	NM210	Have difficulty walking
14.	SKIN203	Itchy skin
15.	SKIN204	Perspire a great deal
16.	CVR202	Frequently feel heart pounding
17.	CVR204	Frequently feel short of breath
18.	CVR209	Frequent dizzy spells
19.	CVR210	Often feel like fainting
20.	CVR213	Frequently feel hot and flushed

mean = 5.565
S.D. = 4.04
K-R 20 reliability = .8234

TABLE 3.

Demographic Characteristics of 255 Women From McKay-Dee Hospitals, All 2nd Trimester

Age	Mean	23.302
	Standard Deviation	4.159
	N	255.000
Marital status	Single	5
	Married	246
	Divorced / Separated	3
	Missing Data	1
		255
Number of children born alive	0	151
	1	53
	2	34
	3	9
	4	5
	·5	3
Was this pregnancy planned?	No	78
	Yes	174
	Missing Data	3
Occupation of head of household (3 Modes)	Professional, including college student	49
	Craftsman	30
	Other, service worker	39

TABLE 4.

Relations of PIPAS Measurement System to 2nd Trimester Symptoms

Initial Preliminary Study

Independent Measure	Dependent Measure I Total 2nd Trimester Symptoms (N=229)
Schedule of recent experience	.37

Final Preliminary Study

	Total 2nd Trimester Symptoms (N=255)	Stress Sensitive Symptom Scale, 2nd Trimester (N=255)
STAGE I		
Social stress	.2716	.2526
Work stress	.1964	.2371
Family stress	.3603	.3583
Financial stress	.2298	.2383
Life style stress	.2617	.2840
Personal habit stress	.4118	.4517
STAGE II		
Regression equation of stresses	.4477	.4835
STAGE III		
Regression equation of stress index and symptom proneness index	.5574	.5672
STAGE IV		
Regression equation of stress index, symptom proneness and Cornell Psychiatric Index (general illness predisposition index)	.7095	.7328
PERCENT VARIANCE EXPLAINED	(50%)	(54%)

TABLE 5.

Partial Correlations Controlling for Family Lifestyle, and Personal Habit Change Stresses

	Total 2nd Trimester Symptoms (N=250)	SIV220 (N=250)
Social stress	.0218 (NS)	.0653 (NS)
Work stress	.0484 (NS)	.0879 (P .082)
Financial Stress	.0261 (NS)	.0249 (NS)

NS = not significant with a single tailed significance level.

APPENDIX C

Stressors and Buffers

During the course of our research we analyzed data in which the effects of buffer variables on stresses were particularly striking. These data came from a Master of Science thesis of Ms. Ann Foster, R.N., conducted under our general supervision.

The thesis problem, essentially, was to determine simple correlations between our stress measures with another stress index on preschool children, which had been conducted by Cottingham and his associates (Cottingham, 1972). Both Cottingham's scale and ours had been developed from the *Schedule of Recent Experience* (SRE). Since these tests had the SRE as an ancestor, it was reasonable to assume that there would be some correlation between them. Inasmuch as the Cottingham scale was a measure of stress on preschoolers and the Utah Stress Scales were measures of stresses on mothers, the scientific problem was to determine the relations of stresses on mothers to stresses on preschoolers. In other words, does a stressed mother tend to have a stressed child, as measured by the two instruments we were using? In trying to answer this problem, we were forced to consider the effects of variables which buffered the effects of stress, and to try to isolate them and to deal with them statistically so the relations of mother to child stresses would be presented in an uncomplicated form.

The following steps were taken in the analysis:

1. Correlations were computed between all the stresses on the mother for the last year and the total stresses on the child. These correlations are in Table 1.
2. A multiple regression equation was computed with child stresses as the dependent variable and the mother's stress scores as the independent variables. With this regression equation with its weights on all the stresses, a stress index was computed.
3. The Stress Index was then combined with age, income, years of education, the Cornell Psychiatric Item Index, and Marital Status (coded as unmarried, married). The relative contribution of each of these variables to the predicted Cottingham score is given by the following equation:

Predicted Cottingham Score = .55426*Mother Stresses — .19567*Marital Status — .12381*Age of Mother — .06959*Education of Mother + .03658*Income — .01837*Cornell Psychiatric Index

The major contributor is stress, with the other variables with a minus loading counteracting the stress. As the values of these variables increases, they reduce the effect of stress. The income variable also covaries with the stress, which would tend to mean that of the stresses we are measuring, when the criterion is preschooler stress index. Increasing income slightly increases the stress. We shall discuss this in a longer report.

4. We took those negatively loaded variables, added them together, and got a new variable called BUFFER. A BUFFER index was computed for each woman and a distribution of these scores was made. The distribution was then split into three groups: Group I = low buffer effect, Group II = medium buffer effect, and Group III = high buffer effect. A high buffer has a strong effect counteracting stresses.
5. Correlations were made between the Cottingham Stress of Preschoolers Index and each of the stress scales, and the total stress index for each of the three groups. Group I, which had the lower buffers, should show a lower correlation of stresses of mothers to stresses of preschoolers. Table 2 shows how the correlations changed from the low to the high buffer group.

We note that our index STRESS, which is the optimum combination of stresses of the mother, has general correlation of .5885 with stresses of preschoolers. For the group that has strong buffering action the correlation is .7432; with weak buffering the relation drops to .4335. In terms of Cottingham Scores we found the following:

	Average Stress on Preschoolers
Group with Stresses Highly Buffered	139.118
Group with Medium Buffered Stresses	185.457
Group with Low Buffering	228.706

We believe that we have demonstrated the stress buffers, their effect when high and low, on the relations of Utah Stress Scales on the mother to the Cottingham Stress Scale on preschoolers. We are most gratified at developing a methodology that demonstrates what we have been talking about clinically for some time but whose effects we had not actually demonstrated statistically, namely, the effect on stresses of buffering variables.

Two findings were interesting. The first was that in the highly buffered group Family Stress had a surprisingly high correlation (.80). The result is that this group of people are relatively insulated from other socioeconomic stresses but not from family stress. The second was that the average correlation of our stress scales and the Cottingham Scale of Mother Stress was highest in the highly buffered group.

TABLE 1.

Correlations of Utah Stress Scales on 98 Mothers with Total Stress Scores on Cottingham Preschool Stress Inventory, 1977

Stresses Over Period 0-12 Months	Correlation With Cottingham Scale
Social stress	.4333
Work stress	.3626
Family stress	.5273
Financial stress	.2530
Life style stress	.5043
Personal stress	.6086

TABLE 2.

	Low Buffer (N=34)	Normal Correlation (N=98)	High Buffer (N=34)
Social stress	.0172	.4333	.5745
Work stress	.2048	.3626	.3480
Family stress	.4656	.5273	.7964
Financial stress	.2849	.2530	.4062
Life style stress	.4607	.5046	.4942
Personal stress	.4971	.4777	.2517
Mother stress	.4335	.6086	.7432
Average correlation	.3377	.4524	.5163

Appendix D

Coping Strategies of Pregnant Women

This series of researches we consider to be interesting failures. They are interesting because in the beginning they seemed to be reasonable ways to open up the important problem of how pregnant women cope with the problems of pregnancy. Furthermore, although not particularly useful for predicting pregnancy symptoms or outcomes, these researches have both developed considerably our conceptions of the problems of pregnant women and have had useful spin-offs. Because there were not substantial studies on pregnancy stress coping, our original theories of this process were constructed on the analogy with processes which psychologists conceptualize interpersonal behaviors. As a result of the work reported here we now conceptualize the coping process of pregnant women based upon the study of successful and unsuccessful adaptations of these women to pregnancy.

The basic model with which we conceptualize the problems of pregnant women is illustrated in Figure 1. The ideas embodied in this model are fairly commonplace. We are primarily concerned with both the infant outcomes of pregnancy and maternal postpartum adaptation. The immediate determiners of these are the course of the labor and delivery. Labor and delivery course, in turn, has an antecedent the symptom course of pregnancy. At this point we introduced the biosocial extensions of the usual research on the pregnancy cycle. We think that the problems of the pregnancy will be due to (a) general reproductive capacity, (b) the pregnancy process and its physiologic load, (c) the social stress load, and (d) an illness or symptom vulnerability of the woman. Illness vulnerability and general reproductive capacity, we assume, will probably depend jointly upon genetic factors and the social, health, and reproductive history of women. Although the model is conventional, the problems of working it out are unconventionally difficult and require the development of a measurement system. Here we discuss our exploratory attempts to develop a set of measures to assess the pregnant woman's appraisal/coping with the pregnancy process.

Our attempt to develop pregnancy appraisal/coping measures was stimulated by and in cooperation with Dr. Mary Manderino, Dr. John Sullivan, Nancy Madsen, and Lois Sullivan. Dr. Manderino had recently completed a Ph.D. dissertation on assertiveness training, a training procedure that we looked upon as almost a universal solvent of personal problems of women. There were three main behaviors that were strengthened in the assertiveness training procedure: (a) asking for changes in the behavior of someone, (b) refusing requests of someone who was asking you to do something you did not wish to do, and (c) giving positive and negative feedback to someone about your feelings. Dr. Manderino had used an unpublished scale of 90 items by Lawrence in her research. This scale had not only poor psychometric properties but also a conceptualization of assertiveness behavior that did not have clearly scorable alternative patterns of social adaptation. The team composed of Mandarino, Madsen, and the Sullivans set up a matrix in which there were five response modes and three situation modes. Typical items of this scale are as follows:

1. A friend asks you to accept a gift that you do not want.
   a. Accept the gift but feel somewhat uncomfortable about doing so.
   b. Accept the gift but indicate you really don't want it.
   c. Accept the gift in order to save your friend embarrassment.
   d. Thank your friend but explain that you cannot accept this gift.
   e. Do not accept the gift.

2. A co-worker sitting next to you in the office indulges in loud gum-chewing all day long every day. This is getting on your nerves.
   a. Ignore her since gum-chewing is a good release for tension.
   b. Tell her to stop chewing gum.
   c. Ask her politely to please chew more quietly.
   d. Tease her about her constant chewing.
   e. Move to the next office.

With the scoring procedure we were able to obtain a score for each individual on Direct Aggression, Indirect Aggression, Assertiveness, Social Compliance, and Passivity and, in addition, we could score the assertive responses into the three categories of Refusing Requests, Asking for Changes in Behavior, and Giving Positive and Negative Feedback. The reliabilities and intercorrelations of these scales are found on Tables 1 and 2, respectively.

Table 3 gives the correlations between these scales and the scales for symptoms each trimester, illness-proneness, and *The Cornell Psychiatric Index*. The striking finding is that the poorest scale psychometrically, the *Direct Aggression Scale,* was significantly correlated with the reports of symptoms during the second trimester. We interpret this finding in two ways: (a) this may be the result of a low socioeconomic crisis life cycle, which is generally associated with increased symptoms; and/or (b) people who are directly aggressive are in an environment that is more stressful, and contribute to this stressful environment in such ways that they tend to have (report) more pregnancy symptoms. The facts that the scales, both the symptoms and the PSA, were highly reliable and that the survey was based upon 237 subjects lead us to the inescapable conclusion that there are few and small relations between our measures and reports of symptoms.

Although the PSA scales did not correlate significantly with the pregnancy symptoms scales, the situation is otherwise with regard to correlations with *The Cornell Psychiatric Index.* From Table 3 it can be seen that the Indirect Aggression Scale correlates significantly in a negative direction with the CPI. This makes sense in terms of our broad conceptualization that assertive management of interpersonal relations will be less associated with depressive/psychotic pathology, which the CPI scale presumable measures.

From the findings of Table 3 it may be said that indirect aggression, passivity, and direct aggression as they are measured by the PSA are associated slightly with psychological pathology as it is measured by the CPI. Furthermore, making requests for changes in behaviors are least associated with pathology which giving positive or negative feedback are more associated with psychological pathology. We suspect, to be consistent with the finding that direct aggression is significantly associated with symptoms, that the correlation of giving positive or negative feedback with the CPI is mainly due to giving negative feedback. If we were to milk these slender findings to a limit we would hypothesize that (a) least pathology is associated with requesting changes in behaviors, and (b) most pathology is associated with giving negative feedback, and (c) intermediate between these alternatives is refusing requests. We do not take these hypotheses very seriously and, furthermore, beliee that they might be rather specific to the situation of young pregnant women in the Intermountain West.

Our internal (within the PIPAS Project) critique of this series of researches was as follows: We had to start somewhere in researching how pregnant women coped with the social, psychological, and physiological load of pregnancy. There were no systematic studies of which we were aware and no systematic insights of the clinicians that were tangible enough to be usable. The result was that we constructed general notions of assertiveness and by analogy tried to deduce how the pregnant woman appraised and coped with her problems. The scales constructed were only successful in a limited way in terms of measurement criteria. This immediately put a limitation on what could possibly come out of the use of such scales.

FIGURE 1. BASIC MODEL OF FACTORS INFLUENCING THE COURSE OF PREGNANCY

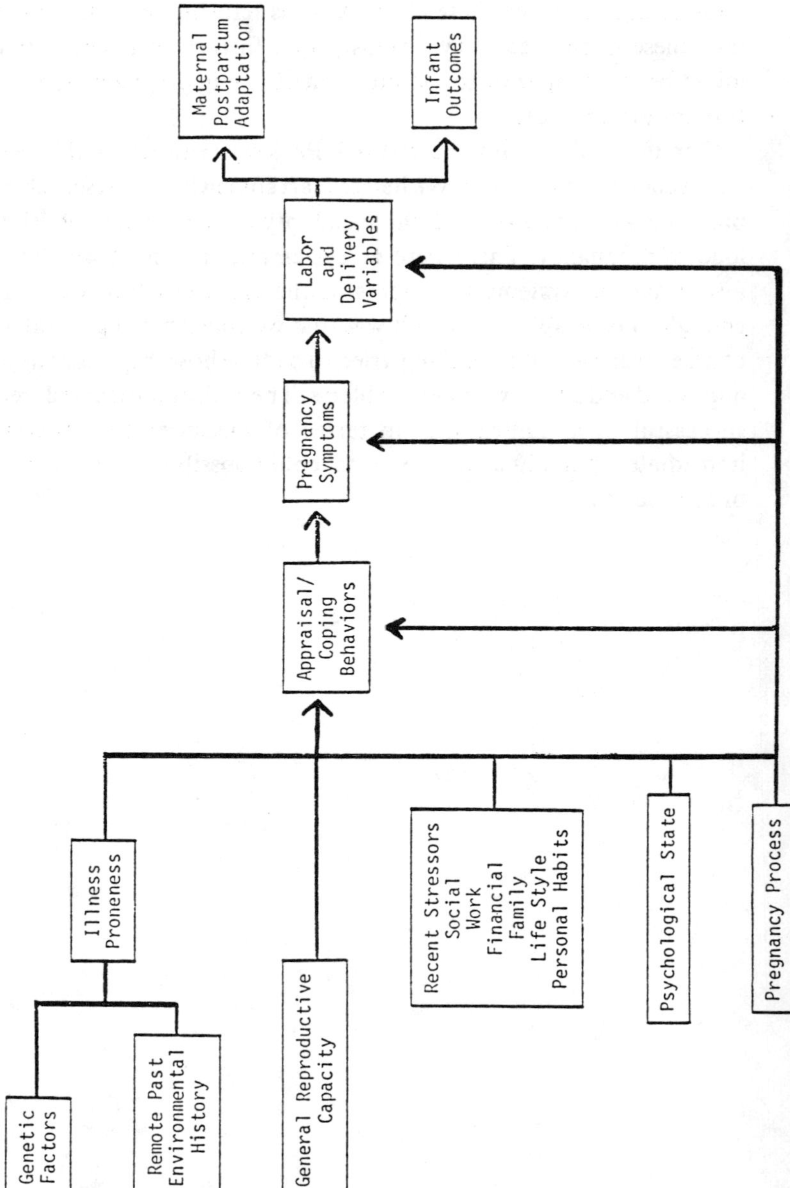

Appendix D

TABLE 1.

Reliabilities of the Scales of the Patterns of Social Adaption Baded Upon 232 Women of Prenatal Classes at McKay-Dee Hospital

Scale	Number of Items	Alpha Reliability
Direct Aggression	31	.6092
Indirect aggression	46	.7932
Assertiveness	87	.9148
Socially compliant	92	.7463
Passive	82	.8623
Making requests for change of behavior	27	.7027
Refusing requests	25	.5620
Giving positive or negative feedback	25	.6278

TABLE 2.

Intercorrelations of Scales of Patterns of Social Adaptation Based Upon 232 Women of Prenatal Classes of McKay-Dee Hospital

Scales	Direct Aggression	Indirect Aggression	Asser-tiveness	Socially Compliant	Passive	Making Requests	Refusing Requests	Feedback
Direct aggression	----	.24	-.08	-.14	-.08	-.01	-.06	-.14
Indirect aggression		----	-.52	.13	.48	-.46	-.38	-.50
Assertiveness			----	-.66	-.82	.91	.87	.90
Socially compliant				----	.52	-.65	-.60	-.56
Passive					----	-.80	-.66	-.74
Making requests for change of behavior							.68	.74
Refusing requests							----	.71
Giving positive or negative feedback								----

TABLE 3.

PM Correlations of Scales of Patterns of Social Adaptation with Symptoms Each Trimester, Illness Proneness, and Cornell Psychiatric Index, of 237 Women in Prenatal Classes, McKay-Dee Hospital

	First Trimester Symptoms	Second Trimester Symptoms	Third Trimester Symptoms	Symptom-Proneness Index	Cornell Psychiatric Index
Direct aggression	.10	.23**	.14*	.05	.14*
Indirect aggression	-.02	.04	-.02	.10	.28*
Assertiveness	-.06	-.03	-.02	-.02	-.25**
Socially compliant	.09	-.03	.07	-.02	.03
Passive	.04	-.03	-.01	-.05	.21**
Making requests for change of behavior	.03	-.05	-.01	-.08	.08
Refusing requests	.00	.00	.01	.11	.17*
Giving positive or negative feedback	.00	-.05	-.07	.07	.21**

* Significant at .05 level.
** Significant at .01 level.

APPENDIX E

TABLE 1

Comparison of Responses to Individual Items in the Domain: Fear of the Childbirth Process, by a General Population Sample from Sale Lake and Weber Counties and Utah Pregnant Primigravid Women

Numbers Used in Questionnaires:			General Population N=382[a] Subjects				Utah Pregnant Primigravidas N=254[a] Subjects			
			Agree		Disagree		Agree		Disagree	
Initial	Final	Item	N	%[b]	N	%[b]	N	%[b]	N	%[b]
11	90	The labor and delivery process is a life-threatening event for the baby.	172	45[c]	207	54	103	41[c]	144	57
29	44	Giving birth is a very pleasant experience.	227	59	152	40[c]	172	68	77	30[c]
39	52	I think I could handle the discomforts of normal labor and delivery without medication.	233	61	142	37[c]	148	58	100	39[c]

TABLE 1 *Continued*

Numbers Used in Questionnaires:			General Population N=382[a] Subjects				Utah Pregnant Primigravidas N=254[a] Subjects			
			Agree		Disagree		Agree		Disagree	
Initial	Final	Item	N	%[b]	N	%[b]	N	%[b]	N	%[b]
40	13	When I think about it, I worry about the pain of labor.	164	43[c]	213	56	171	67[c]	79	31
43	92	Most women I know dread going through childbirth.	124	33[c]	257	67	112	44[c]	139	54
44	74	Few women can cope with the pain of labor without medication.	168	44[c]	211	55	107	42[c]	144	57
55	88	There are often breakdowns in the body's ability to birth a child.	246	64[c]	133	35	103	41[c]	147	58[c]

TABLE 1 *Continued*

Numbers Used in Questionnaires:			General Population N=382[a] Subjects				Utah Pregnant Primigravidas N=254[a] Subjects			
			Agree		Disagree		Agree		Disagree	
Initial	Final	Item	N	%[b]	N	%[b]	N	%[b]	N	%[b]
66	73	It is unusual for the mother to suffer physical damage during the process of normal childbirth.	267	70	112	29[c]	168	66	82	32[c]
88	20	Labor is essentially an unpleasant experience.	164	43[c]	217	57	98	39[c]	150	59
93	53	For the safest labor and delivery a woman should go to an obstetrician.	231	61[c]	147	39	174	69[c]	77	30
100	3	Childbirth is an exprience to be endured.	185	48[c]	194	51	114	45[c]	137	54
103	38	My female family members say labor is difficult and painful.	210	55[c]	169	44	150	59[c]	103	41

TABLE 1 *Continued*

Numbers Used in Questionnaires:			General Population N=382[a] Subjects				Utah Pregnant Primigravidas N=254[a] Subjects			
			Agree		Disagree		Agree		Disagree	
Initial	Final	Item	N	%[b]	N	%[b]	N	%[b]	N	%[b]
116	6	It is unusual for damage to the mother or baby to occur during childbirth.	261	68	118	31[c]	145	57	106	42[c]
120	96	I wish there was some way to have childbirth without any discomfort at all.	253	66[c]	123	32	162	54[c]	89	35
127	37	Childbirth without fear is an unrealistic idea.	144	38[c]	237	62	111	44[c]	142	56
134	51	Childbirth is a safe experience for the mother.	261	68	117	31[c]	144	57	105	41[c]

TABLE 1 *Continued*

Numbers Used in Questionnaires: Initial	Final	Item	General Population N=382[a] Subjects: Agree N	Agree %[b]	Disagree N	Disagree %[b]	Utah Pregnant Primigravidas N=254[a] Subjects: Agree N	Agree %[b]	Disagree N	Disagree %[b]
137	63	Labor and delivery is a necessary evil in order to have a child.	128	34[c]	249	65	77	30[c]	175	69
141	45	Most women are really frightened at the thought of going through labor and delivery.	269	70[c]	112	29	211	83[c]	41	16
151	76	Labor is an exciting experience.	300	79	79	21[c]	196	77	52	20[c]
155	31	The labor and delivery process is one of the most extrfeme physical stresses a woman has in her life.	312	82[c]	69	18	226	69[c]	25	10

TABLE 1 *Continued*

Numbers Used in Questionnaires:			General Population N=382[a] Subjects				Utah Pregnant Primigravidas N=254[a] Subjects			
			Agree		Disagree		Agree		Disagree	
Initial	Final	Item	N	%[b]	N	%[b]	N	%[b]	N	%[b]
171	87	Being in labor is being in a very helpless condition.	140	37[c]	239	63	91	36[c]	154	61

[a]Individual items may have fewer than 382 or 254 responses.

[b]Rounded percents.

[c]Indicates scored direction for both groups of subjects, i.e., toward fear of the childbirth process.

TABLE 2

Comparison of Responses to Individual Items in the Domain: Childbearing Health Locus of Control, by a General Population from Salt Lake and Weber Counties and Utah Pregnant Primigravid Women

Numbers Used in Questionnaires:			General Population N=382[a] Subjects				Utah Pregnant Primigravidas N=254[a] Subjects			
			Agree		Disagree		Agree		Disagree	
Initial	Final	Item	N	%[b]	N	%[b]	N	%[b]	N	%[b]
		Internality:								
152	27	Even though it is difficult to arrange, I can have the kind of childbearing experience I want.	318	83	62	16[c]	212	83	37	15[c]
73	29	I can reduce or eliminate painful sensations during labor by what I do whenever they occur.	328	86	52	14[c]	212	83	35	14[c]

TABLE 2 *Continued*

Numbers Used in Questionnaires:			General Population N=382[a] Subjects				Utah Pregnant Primigravidas N=254[a] Subjects			
			Agree		Disagree		Agree		Disagree	
Initial	Final	Item	N	%[b]	N	%[b]	N	%[b]	N	%[b]
89	1	Women who are prepared to work actively with the labor and delivery process will have an easier child-birth.	364	05	17	5[c]	240	94	13	5[c]
25	32	If I commit myself to active participation during child-birth I will have a much easier experience.	340	89	40	11[c]	240	94	11	4[c]
115	22	My personal health prac-tices are the best means of influencing the outcome of pregnancy.	362	96	16	4[c]	239	94	10	4[c]

TABLE 2 *Continued*

Numbers Used in Questionnaires:			General Population N=382[a] Subjects				Utah Pregnant Primigravidas N=254[a] Subjects			
			Agree		Disagree		Agree		Disagree	
Initial	Final	Item	N	%[b]	N	%[b]	N	%[b]	N	%[b]
109	17	A woman can avoid most complications of pregnancy by what she does to take care of herself.	350	92	28	7[c]	222	87	29	11[c]
		Externality: Powerful Others								
35	33	It is best if I just follow whatever my doctor's or midwife's usual practices are in labor and delivery.	212	56[c]	167	44	147	58[c]	106	42
80	55	It is best to leave the decisions about maternity care to the professionals.	138	36[c]	239	63	114	45[c]	139	55

TABLE 2 *Continued*

Numbers Used in Questionnaires:			General Population N=382[a] Subjects				Utah Pregnant Primigravidas N=254[a] Subjects			
			Agree		Disagree		Agree		Disagree	
Initial	Final	Item	N	%[b]	N	%[b]	N	%[b]	N	%[b]
24	49	I basically trust the competence of physicians during pregnancy and would follow their advice without question.	185	48[c]	271	71	143	56[c]	108	43
156	56	During the childbearing period I should do what my doctor or midwife tells me to regardless of my personal preferences.	108	28[c]	271	71	58	23[c]	192	76
3	69	In order to have a good labor and delivery experience I need to go along with the desires of those in charge of care.	182	48[c]	197	52	144	57[c]	105	41

TABLE 2 *Continued*

Numbers Used in Questionnaires: Initial	Final	Item	General Population N=382[a] Subjects: Agree N	Agree %[b]	Disagree N	Disagree %[b]	Utah Pregnant Primigravidas N=254[a] Subjects: Agree N	Agree %[b]	Disagree N	Disagree %[b]
32	12	The woman and her partner are mostly submissive to the doctor's wishes during childbearing.	244	64[c]	137	36	157	62[c]	92	36
104	81	I depend on experts to tell me most of what I need to know about caring for my body.	175	46[c]	204	53	116	46[c]	136	54
150	95	Just being in the hospital for childbirth would make me feel safe.	245	64[c]	135	35	192	76[c]	60	24

TABLE 2 *Continued*

Numbers Used in Questionnaires: Initial	Final	Item	General Population N=382[a] Subjects: Agree N	Agree %[b]	Disagree N	Disagree %[b]	Utah Pregnant Primigravidas N=254[a] Subjects: Agree N	Agree %[b]	Disagree N	Disagree %[b]
		Externality: Fate/Change								
146	66	It is good luck if I have an easy time during childbearing.	66	17[c]	314	82	71	28[c]	180	71
74	11	Most of the common discomforts during pregnancy just have to be endured as there really isn't anything much to relieve them.	153	40[c]	226	59	136	54[c]	115	45
76	50	Some women are just fated to have complications with childbearing.	131	34[c]	248	59	111	44[c]	139	55

TABLE 2 *Continued*

Numbers Used in Questionnaires:			General Population N=382[a] Subjects				Utah Pregnant Primigravidas N=254[a] Subjects			
			Agree		Disagree		Agree		Disagree	
Initial	Final	Item	N	%[b]	N	%[b]	N	%[b]	N	%[b]
159	70	A baby growth and development is largely due to factors beyond the parents control.	42	11[c]	335	88	34	13[c]	219	86
121	80	I can't do anything to influence the labor and delivery process.	22	6[c]	360	94	24	9[c]	221	87
63	57	There is nothing I can personally do to reduce pain during birth.	20	6[c]	359	94	24	9[c]	226	89

[a]Individual items may have fewer than 382 or 254 responses.

[b]Rounded percents.

[c]Indicates scored direction for both groups of subjects, i.e., toward externality.

TABLE 3

Comparison of Responses to Individual Items in the Domain: Personal Values About Childbearing and Childrearing, by a General Population Sample from Salt Lake and Weber Counties and Utah Pregnant Primigravid Women

Numbers Used in Questionnaires:			General Population N=382[a] Subjects				Utah Pregnant Primigravidas N=254[a] Subjects			
			Agree		Disagree		Agree		Disagree	
Initial	Final	Item	N	%[b]	N	%[b]	N	%[b]	N	%[b]
38	30	Being a mother (father) is one of my most important personal goals.	273	72	108	28[c]	228	90	22	9[c]
145	14	A baby in the family makes it a better functioning unit.	175	46	203	53[c]	152	60	96	38[c]
149	85	The value of being a parent is over-rated.	87	23[c]	291	76	20	8[c]	229	90

TABLE 3 *Continued*

Numbers Used in Questionnaires: Initial	Final	Item	General Population N=382[a] Subjects: Agree N	Agree %[b]	Disagree N	Disagree %[b]	Utah Pregnant Primigravidas N=254[a] Subjects: Agree N	Agree %[b]	Disagree N	Disagree %[b]
170	18	The greatest personal growth in life occurs by being a parent.	183	48	194	51[c]	208	82	41	16[c]
98	34	I don't like the way a baby can tie a couple down.	87	23[c]	292	76	26	10[c]	227	89
144	42	I do not (would not) enjoy routine caretaking of an infant.	80	21[c]	300	79	14	6[c]	238	94
169	54	I've looked forward to having my own baby ever since I was a small child.	198	52	179	47[c]	197	78	56	22[c]

TABLE 3 *Continued*

Numbers Used in Questionnaires: Initial	Final	Item	General Population N=382[a] Subjects: Agree N	%[b]	Disagree N	%[b]	Utah Pregnant Primigravidas N=254[a] Subjects: Agree N	%[b]	Disagree N	%[b]
84	21	Having a baby strengthens a marriage.	195	51	183	48[c]	174	69	78	31[c]
5	67	I have mixed feelings about being a parent.	194	51[c]	186	49	139	55[c]	113	44
122	83	Being a good parent is worthwhile because it is part of God's plan.	288	75	90	24[c]	219	86	28	11[c]
75	5	Husband and wife relationships become closer because of pregnancy.	263	69	114	30[c]	214	84	37	15[c]
164	100	Being a parent does not help you to become a more mature person.	171	45[c]	209	55	93	37[c]	158	62

TABLE 3 *Continued*

Numbers Used in Questionnaires:			General Population N=382[a] Subjects				Utah Pregnant Primigravidas N=254[a] Subjects			
			Agree		Disagree		Agree		Disagree	
Initial	Final	Item	N	%[b]	N	%[b]	N	%[b]	N	%[b]
154	43	Having a baby of your own makes you complete as a woman (man).	94	25	285	75[c]	129	51	123	48[c]
20	19	Having a child gives me (would give me) a sense of living on after I am dead.	174	46	206	54[c]	167	66	84	33[c]
61	68	There isn't much social status in being a mother.	94	25[c]	286	75	48	19[c]	205	81

[a]Individual items may have fewer than 3823 or 254 responses.

[b]Rounded percents.

[c]Indicates scored direction for both groups of subjects, i.e., toward low values.

TABLE 4

Comparison of Responses to Individual Items in the Domain: Father's Role and Responses in Childbearing, by a General Population Sample from Salt Lake and Weber Counties and Utah Pregnant Primigravid Women

Numbers Used in Questionnaires:			General Population N=382[a] Subjects				Utah Pregnant Primigravidas N=254[a] Subjects			
			Agree		Disagree		Agree		Disagree	
Initial	Final	Item	N	%[b]	N	%[b]	N	%[b]	N	%[b]
142	9	A woman needs the sustaining presence of her husband in order to function successfully during labor.	141	37	240	63[c]	170	67	83	33[c]
165	4	Support from her husband is not an essential factor in a woman's ability to successfully control painful sensations during labor.	185	48	194	51	39	15[c]	212	83

TABLE 4 *Continued*

Numbers Used in Questionnaires:			General Population N=382[a] Subjects				Utah Pregnant Primigravidas N=254[a] Subjects			
			Agree		Disagree		Agree		Disagree	
Initial	Final	Item	N	%[b]	N	%[b]	N	%[b]	N	%[b]
140	26	The absence of the expectant father will not affect the successful functioning of a woman during her labor.	163	43[c]	217	57	74	29[c]	177	70
106	28	A woman could not go through labor as successfully without her husband's effort.	222	58	156	41[c]	178	70	72	28[c]
36	35	The expectant father's involvement is not an essential factor in a positive childbirth experience for the woman.	96	27[c]	264	73	46	18[c]	206	81

TABLE 4 *Continued*

Numbers Used in Questionnaires:			General Population N=382[a] Subjects				Utah Pregnant Primigravidas N=254[a] Subjects			
			Agree		Disagree		Agree		Disagree	
Initial	Final	Item	N	%[b]	N	%[b]	N	%[b]	N	%[b]
85	41	If she is committed to a particular approach to labor, a woman will be successful whether or not her husband agrees to it.	169	44[c]	211	55	87	34[c]	165	65
161	60	As long as a man is physically present during labor and delivery, it doesn't matter whether or not he is actively involved in helping his wife.	89	23[c]	291	76	38	15[c]	213	84

TABLE 4 *Continued*

Numbers Used in Questionnaires:			General Population N=382[a] Subjects				Utah Pregnant Primigravidas N=254[a] Subjects			
			Agree		Disagree		Agree		Disagree	
Initial	Final	Item	N	%[b]	N	%[b]	N	%[b]	N	%[b]
82	10	Fathers have more positive, loving feelings toward their newborns when they are present at the delivery than when they are not present.	245	64	135	35[c]	208	82	45	17[c]
167	64	Pregnancy is not physically stressful for an expectant father.	103	27[c]	276	72	61	24[c]	191	75
131	72	Men just aren't able to get involved in every detail of a woman's pregnancy.	190	50[c]	180	50	127	50[c]	122	48

TABLE 4 *Continued*

Numbers Used in Questionnaires:			General Population N=382[a] Subjects				Utah Pregnant Primigravidas N=254[a] Subjects			
			Agree		Disagree		Agree		Disagree	
Initial	Final	Item	N	%[b]	N	%[b]	N	%[b]	N	%[b]
22	77	A woman doesn't want her husband to remind her about her health habits and practices during pregnancy.	92	24[c]	286	75	39	15[c]	213	84
26	84	A husband's support has a lot to do with whether his wife does well during her labor and delivery.	325	85	55	14[c]	221	87	31	12[c]
49	65	A woman needs her husband to participate in developing plans for her labor and delivery.	312	82	68	18[c]	230	91	21	8[c]

TABLE 4 *Continued*

Numbers Used in Questionnaires:			General Population N=382[a] Subjects				Utah Pregnant Primigravidas N=254[a] Subjects			
			Agree		Disagree		Agree		Disagree	
Initial	Final	Item	N	%[b]	N	%[b]	N	%[b]	N	%[b]
48	23	Feeling loved and accepted is not a critical factor in a woman's ability to work successfully with her labor and delivery.	64	17[c]	318	83	21	8[c]	230	91
95	71	If a wife wants her husband to be with her during delivery he should be with her.	310	81	71	19[c]	222	87	28	11[c]
130	89	A woman needs her husband's support and protection during pregnancy because she is more vulnerable physically and emotionally.	340	89	40	11[c]	235	93	11	4[c]

TABLE 4 *Continued*

Numbers Used in Questionnaires:			General Population N=382[a] Subjects				Utah Pregnant Primigravidas N=254[a] Subjects			
			Agree		Disagree		Agree		Disagree	
Initial	Final	Item	N	%[b]	N	%[b]	N	%[b]	N	%[b]
13	61	Expectant fathers have a lot of fears and concerns during childbearing.	332	87	47	13[c]	218	86	34	13[c]
14	36	Women want to be held close and cuddled by their husbands during their pregnancy.	314	82	66	17[c]	213	84	39	15[c]
162	98	It is the father's right to attend the birth of his child.	355	93	25	7[c]	247	97	5	2[c]
77	79	Expectant fathers also have increased needs during pregnancy.	353	92	26	7[c]	255	89	21	8[c]

TABLE 4 *Continued*

Numbers Used in Questionnaires:			General Population N=382[a] Subjects				Utah Pregnant Primigravidas N=254[a] Subjects			
			Agree		Disagree		Agree		Disagree	
Initial	Final	Item	N	%[b]	N	%[b]	N	%[b]	N	%[b]
78	78	Expectant fathers should become involved in the childbearing process.	365	96	15	4[c]	244	96	4	2[c]
133	24	A couple should agree about health care decisions made during the child-bearing experience.	368	96	13	3[c]	238	94	11	4[c]
6	94	The expectant father should provide support to his wife during labor.	373	98	8	2[c]	249	98	3	1[c]

TABLE 4 *Continued*

Numbers Used in Questionnaires:			General Population N=382[a] Subjects				Utah Pregnant Primigravidas N=254[a] Subjects			
			Agree		Disagree		Agree		Disagree	
Initial	Final	Item	N	%[b]	N	%[b]	N	%[b]	N	%[b]
17	97	It is important to a pregnant woman to be reassured of her husband's love and acceptance despite her changing body shape.	375	98	6	2[c]	291	99	1	4[c]

[a]Individual items may have fewer than 382 or 254 responses.

[b]Rounded percents.

[c]Indicates scored direction for both groups of subjects, i.e., toward minimal role and response.

TABLE 5

Comparison of Responses to Individual Items in the Domain: Passive Compliance vs. Active Participation in Childbirth Care Decisions, [a] by a General Population Sample from Salt Lake and Weber Counties and Utah Pregnant Primigravid Women

Numbers Used in Questionnaires:			General Population N=382[a] Subjects				Utah Pregnant Primigravidas N=254[a] Subjects			
			Agree		Disagree		Agree		Disagree	
Initial	Final	Item	N	%[b]	N	%[b]	N	%[b]	N	%[b]
91	2	For the safest outcome when you are in labor, you should do exactly what the hospital personnel tell you to do.	236	62[c]	143	37	196	77[c]	57	22
125	39	Women need a lot of medical help for a difficult experience like childbirth.	106	28[c]	274	72	65	26[c]	186	73
28	7	A woman in labor doesn't have much choice except to follow the usual hospital routines.	140	37[c]	240	63	83	33[c]	168	66

TABLE 5 *Continued*

Numbers Used in Questionnaires:			General Population N=382[a] Subjects				Utah Pregnant Primigravidas N=254[a] Subjects			
			Agree		Disagree		Agree		Disagree	
Initial	Final	Item	N	%[b]	N	%[b]	N	%[b]	N	%[b]
62	46	Traditional approaches to managing labor are safest.	107	28[c]	269	70	83	33[c]	169	67
15	62	I would prefer to manage my own health care and use professional help only to assist me when needed.	204	53	176	46[c]	87	34	163	64[c]
65	16	Without a medical or obstetrical problem I am (my) wife is) as capable as any other woman of birthing a child with minimal medical intervention.	287	75	93	24[c]	204	80	46	18[c]

TABLE 5 *Continued*

Numbers Used in Questionnaires:			General Population N=382[a] Subjects				Utah Pregnant Primigravidas N=254[a] Subjects			
			Agree		Disagree		Agree		Disagree	
Initial	Final	Item	N	%[b]	N	%[b]	N	%[b]	N	%[b]
96	58	I try to do exactly what the doctor/midwife tells me to regarding my (my wife's) care.	302	79[c]	71	19	235	93[c]	18	7
102	8	I feel somewhat helpless to modify my (my wife's) physical health during pregnancy.	91	24[c]	218	74	68	27[c]	182	72
139	82	I trust my doctor/midwife to only give me safe medications/herbs during my pregnancy.	297	78[c]	84	22	225	89[c]	26	10

TABLE 5 *Continued*

Numbers Used in Questionnaires:			General Population N=382[a] Subjects				Utah Pregnant Primigravidas N=254[a] Subjects			
			Agree		Disagree		Agree		Disagree	
Initial	Final	Item	N	%[b]	N	%[b]	N	%[b]	N	%[b]
7	47	I see myself more as a follower than as an initiator.	102	27[c]	227	73	125	49[c]	127	50
58	15	I don't really feel comfortable about participating in the processes of pregnancy and childbirth.	65	17[c]	315	83	38	15[c]	212	83
132	40	I feel confident in being able to protect my own interests during childbearing.	339	89	41	11[ccc]	211	83	41	16[c]

TABLE 5 *Continued*

Numbers Used in Questionnaires:			General Population N=382[a] Subjects				Utah Pregnant Primigravidas N=254[a] Subjects			
			Agree		Disagree		Agree		Disagree	
Initial	Final	Item	N	%[b]	N	%[b]	N	%[b]	N	%[b]
16	75	A woman's doctor/midwife is responsible for keeping a woman healthy during her pregnancy.	70	18	309	81[c]	42	17	209	82[c]
107	91	I want to select my own options and choices about how labor and delivery are managed.	341	89	38	10[c]	218	86	34	13[c]
118	59	It is important to me to participate actively in the process of childbirth.	351	92	29	8[c]	235	93	16	6[c]

TABLE 5 *Continued*

Numbers Used in Questionnaires:			General Population N=382[a] Subjects				Utah Pregnant Primigravidas N=254[a] Subjects			
			Agree		Disagree		Agree		Disagree	
Initial	Final	Item	N	%[b]	N	%[b]	N	%[b]	N	%[b]
51	86	There are a number of equally safe but different approaches to managing labor that a woman can choose to use.	357	94	21	6[c]	229	90	22	9[c]
79	99	Teaching people how to give some of their own care during pregnancy may cause more harm than good.	33	9[c]	346	91	20	8[c]	232	91
108	48	Choosing a health care provider should be primarily based on mutual agreement concerning approaches to childbirth care.	354	93	23	6[c]	238	94	13	5[c]

TABLE 5 *Continued*

Numbers Used in Questionnaires:			General Population N=382[a] Subjects				Utah Pregnant Primigravidas N=254[a] Subjects			
			Agree		Disagree		Agree		Disagree	
Initial	Final	Item	N	%[b]	N	%[b]	N	%[b]	N	%[b]
57	25	It is important to question your doctor/midwife until you understand their advice and concern and then decide whether or not to follow it.	351	92	28	7[c]	229	90	20	8[c]
33	93	Since it is the doctor's/midwife's responsibility to manage the birth, it is not necessary for me to know the details about it.	9	2[c]	372	97	6	2[c]	246	97

[a]Individual items may have fewer than 382 or 254 responses.

[b]Rounded percents.

[c]Indicates scored direction for both groups of subjects, i.e., toward compliance and passive involvement.

Appendix F

Studies Utilizing PIPAS and the Utah Test for the Childbearing Year*

1. PIPAS SCALES:

Deneris, A. (1981). *The PIPAS Project: Stress Factors and Physical Symptoms Relating to Premature Delivery.* Unpublished master's thesis.

Foster, T.A. (1977). *The Relationship of Life Stress in Preschool Children and Their Mothers. Unpublished master's thesis.*

Knackstedt, E.A. (1975). Comparative and Correlative Study Among Psychosocial Assets, Life Change Events, Health Predisposition, Illness Proneness and the Prognosis of Pregnancy. Unpublished master's thesis.

Kosmider, S.B. (1973). *An Analysis of Stress Factors and Illness Proneness Related to the Childbearing Year.* Unpublished master's thesis.

Reilly, L.A. (1979). *Toxemia, Illness Proneness and Stress.* Unpublished master's thesis.

Strahn, M.A. (1979). *Patterns of Nausea and Vomiting in First Pregnancies.* Unpublished master's thesis.

2. Utah Test for the Childbearing Year Scales:

Fuchs, D.A. (1981). *Beliefs and Perceptions About Childbirth of Utah First-Time Fathers.* Unpublished master's thesis.

Martinez, Anita. (1983). *Prenatal Care: Attitudes and Trends of Usage Among Mexican-American Women.* Unpublished master's thesis.

Poore, Marta G. & Foster, Joyce Cameron (1985, Winter). *Epidural and No Epidural Anesthesia: Differences between Mothers and Their Experience of Birth. Birth 12* (4).

*Unpublished master's theses available through interlibrary loan from Eccles Health Sciences Library, University of Utah, Salt Lake City, Utah 84112.

INDEX